New Technologies in Spine Surgery

Editors

ADAM S. KANTER
NICHOLAS THEODORE

NEUROSURGERY
CLINICS OF NORTH AMERICA

www.neurosurgery.theclinics.com

Consulting Editors
RUSSELL R. LONSER
DANIEL K. RESNICK

April 2024 • Volume 35 • Number 2

ELSEVIER

1600 John F. Kennedy Boulevard ● Suite 1800 ● Philadelphia, Pennsylvania, 19103-2899

http://www.theclinics.com

NEUROSURGERY CLINICS OF NORTH AMERICA Volume 35, Number 2
April 2024 ISSN 1042-3680, ISBN-13: 978-0-443-13163-9

Editor: Stacy Eastman
Developmental Editor: Akshay Samson

Neurosurgery Clinics of North America (ISSN 1042-3680) is published quarterly by Elsevier Inc., 360 Park Avenue South, New York, NY 10010-1710. Months of issue are January, April, July, and October. Business and Editorial Offices: 1600 John F. Kennedy Blvd., Suite 1800, Philadelphia, PA 19103-2899. Customer Service Office: 11830 Westline Industrial Drive, St. Louis, MO 63146. Periodicals postage paid at New York, NY, and additional mailing offices. Subscription prices are $465.00 per year (US individuals), $499.00 per year (Canadian individuals), $579.00 per year (international individuals), $100.00 per year (US students), $255.00 per year (international students), and $100.00 per year (Canadian students). For institutional access pricing please contact Customer Service via the contact information below. International air speed delivery is included in all *Clinics* subscription prices. All prices are subject to change without notice. **POSTMASTER:** Send address changes to *Neurosurgery Clinics of North America*, Elsevier Periodicals Customer Service, 11830 Westline Industrial Drive, St. Louis, MO 63146. **Customer Service: 1-800-654-2452 (US and Canada). From outside the US and Canada, call: 1-314-453-7041. Fax: 1-314-453-5170. E-mail: JournalsCustomerService-usa@elsevier.com (for print support) and journalsonlinesupport-usa@elsevier.com (for online support).**

Reprints. For copies of 100 or more, of articles in this publication, please contact the Commercial Reprints Department, Elsevier Inc., 360 Park Avenue South, New York, NY 10010-1710. Tel. 212-633-3874; Fax: 212-633-3820; E-mail: reprints@elsevier.com.

Neurosurgery Clinics of North America is covered in *MEDLINE/PubMed (Index Medicus)*, *EMBASE/Excerpta Medica*, and *Current Contents/Clinical Medicine (CC/CM)*.

Contributors

CONSULTING EDITORS

RUSSELL R. LONSER, MD
Professor and Chair, Department of
Neurological Surgery, The Ohio State
University Wexner Medical Center, Columbus,
Ohio

DANIEL K. RESNICK, MD, MS
Professor and Vice Chairman, Program
Director, Department of Neurosurgery,
University of Wisconsin-Madison School of
Medicine and Public Health, Madison,
Wisconsin

EDITORS

ADAM S. KANTER, MD, MS, MBA, FAANS
Chief, Division of Neurosurgery, Executive
Medical Director, Hoag Neurosciences
Institute, Newport Beach, California

**NICHOLAS THEODORE, MS, MD, FAANS,
FACS**
Professor of Neurosurgery, Orthopaedic Surgery
and Biomedical Engineering, Department of
Neurosurgery, Johns Hopkins University School
of Medicine, Baltimore, Maryland

AUTHORS

NITIN AGARWAL, MD
Associate Professor, Department of
Neurological Surgery, University of Pittsburgh
School of Medicine, UPMC Presbyterian,
Pittsburgh, Pennsylvania

CHRISTOPHER P. AMES, MD
Professor, Department of Neurological
Surgery, University of California, San
Francisco, San Francisco, California

TEJ D. AZAD, MD, MS
Neurosurgery Resident, Department of
Neurosurgery, Johns Hopkins Hospital, The
Johns Hopkins University School of Medicine,
Baltimore, Maryland

AUSAF BARI, MD, PhD
Assistant Professor, UCLA Neurosurgery, Los
Angeles, California

JOEL BECKETT, MD, MHS
Assistant Professor, Department of
Neurosurgery, David Geffen School of
Medicine, University of California, Los Angeles,
Los Angeles, California

MEGHANA BHIMREDDY, BA
Candidate, Department of Neurosurgery, The
Johns Hopkins University School of Medicine,
Baltimore, Maryland

BLAKE BOADI, BS
Research Assistant, Department of
Neurosurgery, Weill Cornell Medicine, New
York-Presbyterian Och Spine Hospital, New
York, New York

CHAD A. CARAWAY, MS
Medical Student research member of the
neurosurgery department research team,
Department of Neurosurgery, Johns
Hopkins School of Medicine, Baltimore,
Maryland

JUSTIN P. CHAN, MD
Orthopaedic Surgery Resident, University of
California, Irvine, Orange, California

LOUIS CHANG, MD
Assistant Professor, Department of
Neurosurgery, Johns Hopkins School of
Medicine, Baltimore, Maryland

A. DANIEL DAVIDAR, MBBS
Research Fellow, Department of Neurosurgery, The Johns Hopkins University School of Medicine, Baltimore, Maryland

GALAL A. ELSAYED, MD
Assistant Professor, Weill Cornell Medicine, NewYork-Presbyterian Och Spine Hospital, New York, New York

TIMOTHY J. FLORENCE, MD, PhD
Resident, UCLA Neurosurgery, Los Angeles, California

ROGER HÄRTL, MD
Professor of Neurological Surgery, Department of Neurosurgery, Weill Cornell Medicine, New York-Presbyterian Och Spine Hospital, New York, New York

DANIEL M. HAFEZ, MD, PhD
Assistant Professor, Department of Neurosurgery, Washington University School of Medicine in St. Louis, St Louis, Missouri

ANDREW M. HERSH, AB
Medical Student, Department of Neurosurgery, The Johns Hopkins University School of Medicine, Baltimore, Maryland

PAWEL P. JANKOWSKI, MD, FAANS
Neurosurgeon, Hoag Spine Center, Newport Beach, California

KELLY JIANG, MS
Candidate, Medical Student, Department of Neurosurgery, The Johns Hopkins University School of Medicine, Baltimore, Maryland

KHANATHIP JITPAKDEE, MD
Spine Consultant, Orthopedic Surgeon, Department of Orthopedics, Queen Savang Vadhana Memorial Hospital, Thai Red Cross Society, Si Racha, Chonburi, Thailand

BRENDAN F. JUDY, MD
Neurosurgery Resident, Department of Neurosurgery, Johns Hopkins Hospital, The Johns Hopkins University School of Medicine, Baltimore, Maryland

ROHIT PREM KUMAR, BA
Department of Neurological Surgery, University of Pittsburgh School of Medicine, UPMC Presbyterian, Pittsburgh, Pennsylvania

ARJUN MENTA, BS, MD
Medical Student, Department of Neurosurgery, Johns Hopkins Hospital, The Johns Hopkins University School of Medicine, Baltimore, Maryland

RORY K. J. MURPHY, MD
Neurosurgeon, Department of Neurosurgery, Barrow Neurological Institute, Neuroscience Publications, St. Joseph's Hospital and Medical Center, Phoenix, Arizona

HO LIM PAK, BS
Medical Student, Department of Neurosurgery, Johns Hopkins Hospital, The Johns Hopkins University School of Medicine, Baltimore, Maryland

ANSHUL RATNAPARKHI, BS
Staff Researcher, Department of Neurosurgery, David Geffen School of Medicine, University of California, Los Angeles, Los Angeles, California

SHAHAB ALDIN SATTARI, MD
Postdoctoral Research Fellow, Department of Neurosurgery, Johns Hopkins School of Medicine, Baltimore, Maryland

JUSTIN K. SCHEER, MD
Resident, Department of Neurological Surgery, University of California, San Francisco, San Francisco, California

NICHOLAS THEODORE, MS, MD, FAANS, FACS
Professor of Neurosurgery, Orthopaedic Surgery and Biomedical Engineering, Department of Neurosurgery, Johns Hopkins University School of Medicine, Baltimore, Maryland

ANDREW C. VIVAS, MD
Assistant Professor, UCLA Neurosurgery, Los Angeles, California

CARLY WEBER-LEVINE, MS
Candidate, Medical Student, Department of Neurosurgery, The Johns Hopkins University School of Medicine, Baltimore, Maryland

TIMOTHY F. WITHAM, MD
Professor of Neurosurgery and Orthopaedic Surgery, Department of Neurosurgery, Johns Hopkins Hospital, The Johns Hopkins University School of Medicine, Baltimore, Maryland

YUANXUAN XIA, MD
Resident, Department of Neurosurgery, Johns Hopkins School of Medicine, Baltimore, Maryland

Contents

Advances in Imaging (Intraop Cone-Beam Computed Tomography, Synthetic Computed Tomography, Bone Scan, Low-Dose Protocols)   161

Pawel P. Jankowski and Justin P. Chan

Spine surgery has seen a rapid advance in the refinement and development of 3-dimensional and nuclear imaging modalities in recent years. Cone-beam CT has proven to be a valuable tool for improving the accuracy of pedicle screw placement. The use of synthetic CT and low-dose CT have also emerged as modalities which allow for little to no radiation while streamlining imaging workflows. Bone scans also serve to provide functional information about bone metabolism in both the preoperative and postoperative monitoring phases.

Image-Guided Spine Surgery   173

Khanathip Jitpakdee, Blake Boadi, and Roger Härtl

The realm of spine surgery is undergoing a transformative shift, thanks to the integration of image-guided navigation technology. This innovative system seamlessly blends real-time imaging data with precise location tracking. While the indispensable expertise of experienced spine surgeons remains irreplaceable, navigation systems bring a host of valuable advantages to the operating room. By offering a comprehensive view of the surgical anatomy, these systems empower surgeons to conduct procedures with accuracy, while minimizing radiation exposure for both patients and medical professionals. Moreover, image-guided navigation paves the way for integration of other state-of-the-art technologies, such as augmented reality and robotics. These innovations promise to further revolutionize the field, providing greater precision and expanding the horizons of what is possible in the world of spinal procedures. This article explores the evolution, classification, and impact of image-guided spine surgery, underscoring its pivotal role in enhancing efficacy and safety while setting the stage for the incorporation of future technological advancements.

Functional Stimulation and Imaging to Predict Neuromodulation of Chronic Low Back Pain   191

Timothy J. Florence, Ausaf Bari, and Andrew C. Vivas

Back pain is one of the most common aversive sensations in human experience. Pain is not limited to the sensory transduction of tissue damage; rather, it encompasses a range of nervous system activities including lateral modulation, long-distance transmission, encoding, and decoding. Although spine surgery may address peripheral pain generators directly, aberrant signals along canonical aversive pathways and maladaptive influence of affective and cognitive states can result in persistent subjective pain refractory to classical surgical intervention. The clinical identification of who will benefit from surgery—and who will not—is increasingly grounded in neurophysiology.

poor. Extensive research and ongoing clinical trials seek to design new treatment options for spinal cord injury, including stem cell therapy, scaffolds, brain–spine interfaces, exoskeletons, epidural electrical stimulation, ultrasound, and cerebrospinal fluid drainage. Some of these treatments are targeted at the initial acute window of injury, during which secondary damage occurs; others are designed to help patients living with chronic injuries.

The amount and quality of data being used in our everyday lives continue to advance in an unprecedented pace. This digital revolution has permeated healthcare, specifically spine surgery, allowing for very advanced and complex computational analytics, such as artificial intelligence (AI) and machine learning (ML). The integration of these methods into clinical practice has just begun, and the following review article will describe AI/ML, demonstrate how it has been applied in adult spinal deformity surgery, and show its potential to improve patient care touching on future directions.

Applications and workflows around spinal robotics have evolved since these systems were first introduced in 2004. Initially approved for lumbar pedicle screw placement, the scope of robotics has expanded to instrumentation across different regions. Additionally, precise navigation can aid in tumor resection or spinal lesion ablation. Robot-assisted surgery can improve accuracy while decreasing radiation exposure, length of hospital stay, complication, and revision rates. Disadvantages include increased operative time, dependence on preoperative imaging among others. The future of robotic spine surgery includes automated surgery, telerobotic surgery, and the inclusion of machine learning or artificial intelligence in preoperative planning.

NEUROSURGERY CLINICS OF NORTH AMERICA

SERIES OF RELATED INTEREST

Neurologic Clinics
https://www.neurologic.theclinics.com/
Neuroimaging Clinics
https://www.neuroimaging.theclinics.com/

THE CLINICS ARE AVAILABLE ONLINE!
Access your subscription at:
www.theclinics.com

Preface

Transformative Spine Surgery: A Paradigm Shift in Treatment and Technology

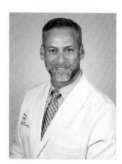   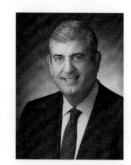

Adam S. Kanter, MD, MS, MBA, FAANS   Nicholas Theodore, MS, MD, FAANS, FACS

Editors

The field of spinal surgery has experienced a surge of transformative advancements, departing from traditional reliance on harvested autografts, stainless steel implants, and continuous fluoroscopy. This issue deals with the latest advances and the future of the field of spinal surgery. The last three decades have been a remarkable journey, showcasing a leap in surgical techniques and approaches that have forever transformed the care of our patients with degenerative, traumatic, neoplastic, and infectious processes.

The integration of enabling technologies, such as image guidance, robotics, intraoperative imaging, and augmented reality, has revolutionized the placement of spinal instrumentation, enhancing both speed and accuracy. Additional refinements in implants are adding to the excitement of improving our fusion rates and ability to reconstruct the spine. Select innovations include advanced surface coating to augment bony ingrowth into nonbiologic materials, expandable constructs, and an enriched understanding of spinal biomechanics and load sharing.

At the cusp of this wave stands the burgeoning potential of artificial intelligence. Its capacity to tailor surgical strategies to individual patient profiles and prognosticate outcomes is a budding expectation that will emerge through iterative evolution. Assessing our patients through the continuum of care will be a critical feature in measuring the prospective benefit of invasive procedures. Furthermore, digital phenotyping, utilizing wearable technologies, promises to redefine our benchmarks for patient improvement.

As we look forward, the field of spinal surgery is advancing at an unprecedented pace, benefiting from the cross-pollination of material science, imaging physics, robotics, and data analysis. Amidst these significant advancements, the spinal surgery community looks to the future with enduring excitement, confident in the promise of continued innovation through transformative patient care.

Adam S. Kanter, MD, MS, MBA, FAANS
Division of Neurosurgery
Hoag Neurosciences Institute
Newport Beach, CA, USA

Nicholas Theodore, MS, MD, FAANS, FACS
Orthopaedic Surgery &
Biomedical Engineering
Department of Neurosurgery
Johns Hopkins University School of Medicine
Baltimore, MD, USA

E-mail addresses:
ak1steelspine@gmail.com (A.S. Kanter)
Theodore@jhmi.edu (N. Theodore)

Neurosurg Clin N Am 35 (2024) ix
https://doi.org/10.1016/j.nec.2024.01.001
1042-3680/24/© 2024 Published by Elsevier Inc.

Advances in Imaging (Intraop Cone-Beam Computed Tomography, Synthetic Computed Tomography, Bone Scan, Low-Dose Protocols)

Pawel P. Jankowski, MD[a],*, Justin P. Chan, MD[b]

KEYWORDS

- Spine imaging • Synthetic CT • Cone beam CT • Bone scan • Low-dose CT

KEY POINTS

- Cone-beam computed tomography (CT) has proved to be a valuable tool during spine surgery to evaluate accuracy of pedicle screw placement while at the same time being utilized for CT-guided navigation of spinal implants.
- Synthetic CT has emerged as a valuable tool in spine surgery, providing accurate, radiation-free, 3-dimensional imaging of bony anatomy and pathology, while streamlining the preoperative workflow with single-modality imaging.
- Low-dose CT scans have emerged as a valuable imaging modality in spine surgery, striking a balance between diagnostic accuracy and minimizing radiation exposure.
- Bone scans serve as valuable tools in spine surgery, providing functional information about bone metabolism and aiding in the diagnosis, surgical planning, and postoperative evaluation of various spinal pathologies.

INTRODUCTION

The field of instrumented spine surgery has seen a steady pace of development in the past 4 decades since the development and adoption of the pedicle screw as a mode of spinal fixation to treat various spine pathologies. In order for a spinal implant such as the pedicle screw to achieve its peak effectiveness, proper placement is needed. The volume of pedicle screws that is being placed in spine surgeries throughout the country has seen a tremendous increase in the past decades due to the increase in spinal fusion procedures being performed. Between 1988 and 2001, rates of lumbar fusion surgery among patients over the age of 60 increased by 230%.[1] Martin and colleagues reported the greatest increase among age 65 and above in lumbar instrumented fusion, increasing 138.7% by volume from 98.3 per 100,000 in 2004 to 170.3 in 2015.[2] This increase also raises the potential for misplaced pedicle screw implants that can result in clinically significant events. Spinal intraoperative navigation techniques that are computed tomography (CT) based have become a critical part of spine surgery nowadays due to their improved accuracy of pedicle screw placement and therefore reduction of misplaced screws compared with conventional

a Hoag Spine Center, 520 Superior Avenue, #300, Newport Beach, CA 92663, USA; b University of California, Irvine, 101 The City Drive South, Orange, CA 92868, USA
* Corresponding author. 16305 Sand Canyon Avenue, Suite 220, Irvine, CA 92618.
E-mail address: Pawel.jankowski@hoag.org

Neurosurg Clin N Am 35 (2024) 161–172
https://doi.org/10.1016/j.nec.2023.11.007
1042-3680/24/© 2023 Elsevier Inc. All rights reserved.

freehand and fluoroscopy techniques.[3–8] Despite pedicle screws being placed on a regular basis, there are challenges that remain for surgeons for the optimal anatomic placement of screws especially in certain spinal pathologies where anatomic landmarks can be difficult to discern. Pedicle screws that are not in the correct position may lead to revision surgeries, increased health care costs, persistent pain, and even neurologic deficits.[1,9,10]

Mobile Versus Non-mobile Intraoperative Computed Tomography Navigation

The 2 most common forms of CT-based image acquisition and navigation in spine surgery currently are sliding gantry (SGCT) and mobile cone-beam CT (CBCT), **Fig. 1**A–C. Both have their advantages and disadvantages relative to each other. The most apparent advantage of CBCT is that it is mobile and can be shuttled between different operating rooms in a hospital. It can perform CT scanning rapidly and be utilized as 2-dimensional fluoroscopy machines simultaneously.[11] SGCTs have a wider field of view which is helpful when imaging the cervicothoracic spine and patients with larger body habitus.[12]

Radiation during spine surgery remains an important factor to consider with the use of these CT navigation units. This includes radiation exposure to the patient and to the surgeon. Factors such as distance from the source, shielding, and fluoroscopy time affect radiation dose.[13] Serious health risks are associated with increased cumulative radiation exposure.[13–16] As a result, minimizing radiation exposure to the patient and staff while not sacrificing accuracy during surgery is important.[13–16] CT-guided navigation platforms that are CBCT and SGCT based offer the advantage over 2D fluoroscopy methods that both the surgeon and operating room staff can leave the room in order to avoid radiation. However, the patient still suffers exposure during this process. Therefore, finding a navigation platform that lowers the cumulative amount of radiation is crucial. In a study by Baumgart and colleagues, they demonstrated that using SGCT-based navigation for pedicle screw placement provides significantly lower radiation exposure to the patient when compared to CBCT.[11] The authors were also able to demonstrate that SGCT had a lower number of intraoperative screw revisions compared to CBCT and showed improved image clarity and therefore lowered cumulative radiation during a procedure due to less need for revision of suboptimal screws.[11]

Validation of Intraoperative Computed Tomography Navigation and Accuracy

In a meta-analysis that compared intraoperative CT-based navigation versus fluoroscopy, intraoperative CT was shown to result in shorter operative time versus fluoroscopy and have significantly lower rates of pedicle screw deviation and perioperative complications.[17] When screws placed using CT-based navigation platforms were compared to freehand pedicle screw insertion, it was demonstrated that the length of surgery was shorter, there was decreased blood loss, decreased overall complications and need for reoperation.[12,18–20]

Cone-Beam Computed Tomography Platforms

A traditional CT scan employs a fan-shaped anode X-ray beam, while CBCT uses a round or rectangular cone-shaped beam with an area detector (vs a linear group of detectors).[21] The CBCT has shorter scan times (approx.. 1 min) while providing high-quality images with sub-millimeter resolution along with high-dimensional accuracy (ie, 3D volumetric data in axial, sagittal, and coronal planes). Furthermore, the radiation that is put out from a standard CBCT module is considerably lower (on the order of 10-fold less) compared to conventional CT scans.[22] However, the levels are not inconsequential and well-exceed daily background amounts of radiation in the natural environment ($\sim$8.2 μSv per day in the United States).[21–23] Furthermore, certain CBCT scanners contain intensified X-ray sources that have drastically higher levels of radiation.

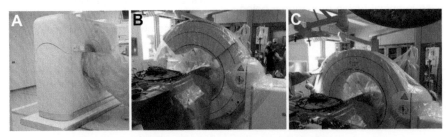

Fig. 1. Sliding gantry computed tomography (CT) (*A*), cone- beam CT (*B, C*).

Differences Between Cone Beam Computed Tomography Systems

Concerning CBCT modules that are in use throughout the world for intraoperative navigation applications in spine surgery, the most widely used is O-armO2 (Medtronic, Minneapolis, MN, USA). Many of the comparative metrics used to assess CBCT modules are based on the O-armO2 performance. Rousseau and colleagues demonstrated that in terms of radiation effective dose (ED), the Surgivisio system (eCential Robotics, Gières, France) showed 5 to 12 times reduction in radiation ED compared to the O-armO2 system during spine procedures.[24] This is in part related to the optimized partial-angle non-isocentric trajectory for CBCT during image acquisition and the low-dosage radiation setting that can be utilized on the Surgivisio system during acquisition of 3D images.[24] Neither system was shown to be adequate for diagnostic purposes, lacking the imaging detail of osseus and soft tissue structures of conventional CT.[24] In a study comparing the O-arm against the Airo (Brainlab AG, Munich, Germany), it was shown that the O-arm had lower contrast-to-noise ratio but improved spatial resolution compared to the Airo.[25] The improved resolution with the usage of high-definition protocols with the O-arm results in 56% larger radiation ED compared to the Airo.[25] The O-arm showed better performance compared to the Airo in regards to pedicle screw positioning in the lumbar spine with better spatial resolution of anatomic features.[25] A new intraoperative mode of CT imaging that maintains the same detail of imaging with applications for navigation of implants without the radiation burden of conventional CT is synthetic CT.

Advances and future directions

Cone-beam CT can be used to assess for instability of the spine. It has the ability to accurately identify any instability through its multi-planar capabilities, which can be quite useful in the presence of surgical hardware.[26] CBCT allows for assessment of flexion and extension of the neural foramina and facet joints in a weight-bearing position and can show the paraspinal muscle volumes and any fatty infiltration.[26] Such detail can be useful in patients with occult back and leg pain where no etiology was identified on static MRI or CT imaging.

Challenges and limitations

The primary limitation of CBCT remains the radiation dose administered to the patient during usage. Although CBCT has an overall lower dose than conventional CT scanning units, the amount is not negligible. Furthermore, anatomic detail and clarity of images generated using SGCT are still lacking compared to conventional CT.

Summary

Cone-beam CT has proved to be a valuable tool during spine surgery to evaluate accuracy of pedicle screw placement while at the same time being utilized for CT- guided navigation of spinal implants. Further refinement of this technology will be focused on decreasing radiation while at the same time improving the imaging detail.

SYNTHETIC COMPUTED TOMOGRAPHY

Spine surgery demands exceptional precision in imaging due to the proximity of critical neural structures within the surgical field and the intricate anatomy of the spine. Detailed preoperative planning is paramount to identify pathology, determine optimal approaches, and plan instrumentation trajectories. Traditional preoperative imaging modalities, such as CT and MRI, are essential for surgical planning but each have inherent limitations. The need for obtaining both types of imaging can lead to delays in surgical intervention as well as significant radiation exposure. MRI allows for very high contrast of soft-tissue and neurologic structures, making it the diagnostic study of choice for the majority of spinal pathologies. It offers high sensitivity and specificity when diagnosing tumors, infections, pathologic fractures, disc degeneration, and herniations. However, when high resolution of the osseus structures is necessary, MRI lacks the detail compared to CT. If neuronavigation is part of the operative procedure, CT images are often required for treatment planning, such as for image-guided navigated biopsies or pedicle screw placement.[27]

CT allows for a detailed depiction of the topogropraphy, geometry, stability, and abnormality of the osseus structures that can affect the placement of implants and manipulation of the spine. Despite the lower cost of CT compared to MRI, multiple imaging sessions increase the burden to the patient, overall costs and introduce complex workflows, with the potential for intermodality registration errors (**Figs. 2**A–D and **3**).[28] Although the greatest disadvantage is the increased ionizing radiation to the patient, which is especially problematic in the pediatric population. The average lumbar spinal CT radiation exposure equals an effective dose of around 3.5 mSv up to 19.5 mSv.[28–33] Therefore, the ability to incorporate osseus detail at the level of a CT in an MRI modality would be advantageous. Synthetic CT is a novel, noncontrast, and rapid MRI method that

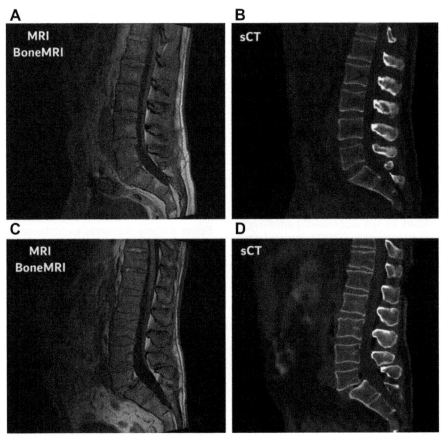

Fig. 2. Scans were first performed on volunteer test subjects to train the MRI algorithm and then on volunteers that were not used as part of the machine learning protocol. Bone MRI sequences acquired in 2 volunteers not represented in the training data set (*A* and *C*), along with the corresponding sCT images generated (*B* and *D*). Midsagittal cuts of the lumbar spine are shown.[28]

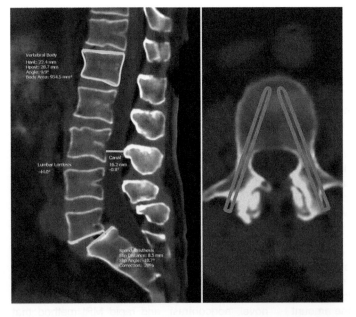

Fig. 3. A midsagittal synthetic computed tomography (CT) cut (*left*) along with an axial reconstruction (*right*). Conventional measurements such as spinal canal diameter, lumbar lordosis, and spondylolisthesis grading (Meyerding grade II) as well as semiautomated measurements such as vertebral body segmentation were carried out. In addition, pedicle screw trajectories and screw thickness for both L5 pedicles were estimated on sCT imaging.[28]

can produce CT-quality images without the radiation exposure of a traditional CT and it is easily performed in conjunction with traditional MRI, which detects soft-tissue and bone marrow abnormalities.[34]

Generation of Synthetic Computed Tomographies

The methods for generating synthetic CTs fall into 3 main categories: atlas based, machine learning, and deep learning.[35] Atlas-based methods use pre-segmented CT atlases to align with the patient's MRI data. The atlas's anatomic information is deformed and adapted to the patient's MRI, generating a synthetic CT image. While effective, atlas-based methods require high-quality atlases and may encounter challenges with individual anatomic variations. Machine learning models, such as convolutional neural networks (CNNs), have demonstrated exceptional promise in generating synthetic CT images. These models are trained on large datasets of paired MRI and CT images, learning to map MRI features to corresponding CT Hounsfield unit values. Machine learning–based approaches improve accuracy and reduce the reliance on atlases. Finally, generative adversarial networks (GANs) are a class of deep learning models that consist of a generator and a discriminator, competing in a game-like framework.[36] The generator creates synthetic CT images, while the discriminator evaluates their realism. This iterative process refines the synthetic CT images until they become indistinguishable from real CT scans, offering high-quality synthetic representations for surgical planning.

Validation and Accuracy of Synthetic Computed Tomography

Recent studies explored generating radiograph-like and CT-like images from MRI scans to improve osseous structure visualization. Gersing and colleagues found that MRI-derived radiograph-like images were feasible for bone tumor evaluation and were comparable to radiographs.[37] Argentieri and Breighner were able to create MRI-based CT-like images based on 0 echo time sequences and reported good agreement with standard CT of the spine and hips.[38,39] However, this qualitative technique lacks specificity for cortical bone and requires specific hardware. In contrast, deep learning–based synthetic CT (sCT) was developed specifically to visualize osseous structures in a quantitative way based on attenuation maps; thus, it can accurately depict cortical and subcortical bone.[40] Meanwhile, postprocessing of sCT

images is a fully automatic process that does not require user input.

The cervical region of the spinal column can still be surgically challenging with current conventional CT navigation. In part, this is due to the difficulty of immobilization during surgery and another due to the vascular and neural structures present in close proximity of the surgery. In a single-center study from the Netherlands, van der Kolk and colleagues were able to demonstrate qualitative assessment of sCT images in study participants with cervical radiculopathy to be noninferior compared to conventional CT in the general depiction of cervical anatomy structures and artifacts.[41]

Morbee and colleagues performed a study to test the equivalence of MRI-based synthetic CT to conventional CT in order to quantitatively assess bony morphology of the lumbar spine (**Fig. 4**A–D).[42] Synthetic CT images were generated from MRI using machine deep learning methods.[42] Thirty participants were included (14 men and 16 women, range 20–60 years). The anatomic measurements performed on sCT were statistically equivalent to conventional CT measurements and there was excellent inter- and intra-reader reliability for both synthetic CT and conventional CT, **Fig. 4**A–D.[42]

The 1 exception has been pedicle measurements in the axial plane, which were shown by 1 study of GAN-based synthetic CTs to be less accurate than conventional CT with a relative error up to 34%.[43,44] While large-scale validation studies have yet to be conducted, the existing literature has so far shown relatively high concordance with conventional CT, supporting the reliability of synthetic CT for surgical planning.

Radiation-Free Surgical Planning

Synthetic CT can also be integrated into navigation systems which can then be registered to the patient based on topographic landmarks, eliminating the need for intraoperative CT scans and fluoroscopy. The ultimate goal of CT navigation platforms in spine surgery is to be able to merge soft tissues, vascular structures, neurologic detail, and osseus features all together in real time during the procedure.

Studies looking at the application of sCT toward surgical navigation and diagnostic goals for the spinal column have demonstrated promising results. Staartjes and colleagues utilizing a research prototype from previous work were able to show that the quality of the generated sCT scans was sufficient for surgical planning and neuronavigation and could even suffice for diagnostic purposes in all the patients in their test group,

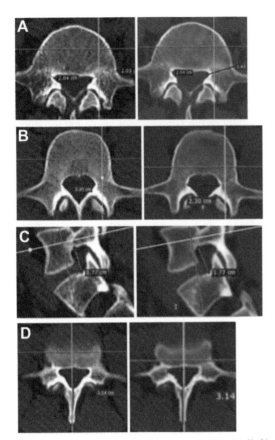

Fig. 4. Same outcome of measurements on CT (*left*) and synthetic CT (*right*). (*A*) Axial images of left and right pedicle of vertebra L5, (*B*) axial images of spinal canal of vertebra L4, (*C*) sagittal images of neuroforamen on level L5-S1, (*D*) axial images of spinous process of vertebra L5.[42]

Figs. 2 and 3.[28,34,40,41,46] **This was a low-volume patient study; however, it demonstrated the advancements in machine learning to provide bony detail in an MRI format without the radiation of a conventional CT scan.**

Advances and Future Directions

The integration of synthetic CT with additional imaging modalities, such as functional MRI and diffusion tensor imaging, holds promise for enhancing surgical planning by providing more comprehensive information about functional neural connectivity and white matter tracts.

Challenges and Limitations

Synthetic CT is still not a perfect substitute for traditional CT. Whereas CT images directly measure radiological characteristics of the tissue, MRI intensities rely on proton density and can result in some ambiguity between bone and air which both appear dark on MRI despite having very different coefficients of attenuation.[47,48] MRI images are also more susceptible to geometric distortions than CT, particularly in the outer edges of the MRI's field of view where the magnetic field becomes increasingly non-linear.[49]

The generation of synthetic CT images can also be computationally intensive, requiring powerful hardware and efficient algorithms to ensure real-time applications during surgery. Machine learning–based approaches are also highly dependent on the quality and diversity of the training datasets. Ensuring comprehensive and representative datasets is critical to achieving accurate synthetic CT generation.

Summary

Synthetic CT has emerged as a valuable tool in spine surgery, providing accurate, radiation-free, 3D imaging of bony anatomy and pathology, while streamlining the preoperative workflow with single-modality imaging. The methods of generating synthetic CT are continuing to be refined, along with its applications in workflow for preoperative planning and intraoperative navigation.

BONE SCAN

Bone scan, also known as bone scintigraphy or single-photon emission computed tomography (SPECT), is a nuclear medicine study which involves using a small amount of radioactive tracer to detect uptake throughout the skeletal system. This allows for valuable information about the metabolic activity of bone. Most bone scans involve the intravenous administration of a radiopharmaceutical, typically technetium-99m (99mTc)-labeled phosphonates combined with a scintillation camera. A gamma camera detects the emitted gamma rays, creating images that visualize the distribution of the radiotracer and revealing areas of increased or decreased bone activity. When applied correctly, bone scans offer unique insights into the pathophysiology of spinal disorders that enhance diagnostic accuracy, guide treatment planning, and monitor patient progress.

Infections and Tumors

Bone scans are highly sensitive in identifying the most metabolically active areas associated with infectious processes. In cases of vertebral osteomyelitis and discitis, bone scans help confirm the diagnosis, delineate the extent of infection, and help inform the appropriate surgical and medical management as well as extent of resection or debridement if necessary, **Fig. 5.**[50]

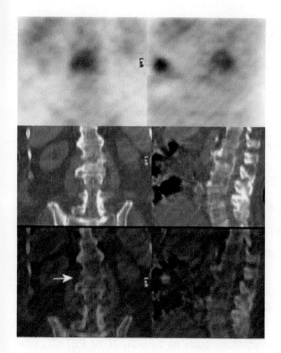

Coronal   Sagittal

Fig. 5. Spinal osteomyelitis. There is increased activity in the upper lumbar spine on the coronal and sagittal ^{67}Ga single-photon emission computed tomography(-SPECT) images (*top*). There is vertebral endplate destruction at the level of L1-L2 on the CT component (*center*). The fused SPECT/CT images (*bottom*) localize the increased ^{67}Ga activity to L1-L2, and demonstrate extension of the abnormal activity into the adjacent soft tissues (*arrow*), which is not apparent on the SPECT images alone (*top*). As this case illustrates, SPECT/CT contributes useful information by precisely localizing radiopharmaceutical uptake and facilitating the identification of soft-tissue involvement by the infection.[50]

Bone scans are also instrumental in detecting and localizing primary and metastatic spinal tumors. By identifying sites of increased bone activity, they can identify optimal locations for targeted biopsies, as well as delineate spinal levels affected by the malignancy. As the field of view for bone scans typically involves the entire body, distant metastases can also be identified at the same time. This can help inform treatment decisions if a cancer is deemed to be isolated to the spine and curable with a wide excision, or for a cancer which has already diffusely metastasized, a more limited palliative decompression may be indicated to relieve spinal cord or nerve root compression. Postoperatively, follow-up bone scans are also valuable for detecting early signs of recurrence or new metastatic spread, allowing for timely treatment adjustments.

Assessing Spinal Fusion

Bone scans also play a vital role in evaluating the success of spinal fusions. Persistent or increasing metabolic activity at the fusion site may indicate non-union or pseudoarthrosis, prompting appropriate intervention, **Fig. 6**.[45] Studies involving serial bone scans of healing posterolateral fusion masses in the lumbar and sacral spine have shown a steady decrease in osteoblastic activity of the fusion mass after 3 months.[51] Persistent radiotracer uptake beyond 1 year after surgery, particularly at the facet joints, may represent continued motion indicative of a pseudarthrosis.[52] It is important to note that the use of bone scans to assess pseudarthrosis 6 months after index surgery has been associated with a 50% false-positive rate, and increased uptake is not necessarily suggestive of pseudarthrosis until 1 year after surgery.[53]

Assessing metabolic activity at adjacent levels can also be valuable in differentiating between natural age-related degeneration and pathologic changes that may require surgical intervention. Heimburger and colleagues reported a sensitivity and specificity of 88.2% and 93.9% for adjacent level degeneration, 80.7% and 82.7% for posterior pseudarthrosis, 100% and 60% for interbody pseudoarthrosis, and 68.2% and 91.7% for hardware loosening, respectively.[54] A study by Evan-Sapir et al. also found abnormal uptake on SPECT scans in the vertebral bodies and apophyseal joints of free motion segments adjacent to fused segments in patients who had undergone fusion surgery more than 4 years prior, compared to early postoperative patients.

Hardware loosening is another aspect of postoperative spinal fusions which can be assessed with bone scans. Pedicle screw loosening is typically associated with pseudarthrosis and may not be detectable on MRI or CT until there is significant motion around a screw, or it pulls out or fractures entirely. A study by Hudynaa and colleagues found that bone SPECT has 100% sensitivity and 89.7% specificity for detecting screw loosening.[55]

Occult Trauma

In cases of occult trauma or insufficiency fractures where conventional radiographs and even CT scans may be inconclusive, bone scans reveal areas of increased activity, guiding further diagnostic workup and potential surgical intervention. This is particularly useful in the case of lumbar spondylolysis in the pediatric population. Plain radiographs are often negative unless there is frank spondylolisthesis. Literature suggests that even with advanced imaging, pars defects are detected in only 32% to 44% of adolescents with spondylolysis. SPECT

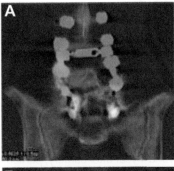
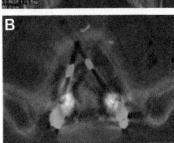
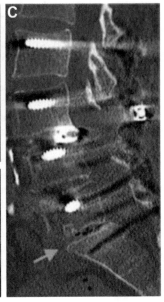

Fig. 6. Pseudarthrosis. Coronal fused SPECT/CT (*A*), axial fused SPECT/CT (*B*), and sagittal CT (*C*) show L2–S1 fusion with increased osteoblastic activity at the L5/S1 facet joints bilaterally (*A*, *B*) and vacuum phenomenon at the L5/S1 disc space (*C*, *arrow*), representing instability at L5/S1.[45]

has been shown to be superior to planar bone scan and plain radiographs although limited in efficacy by high false-positive rates and high radiation dose in a pediatric population.[56] Although conventional CT remains the gold standard for diagnosis of pediatric spondylolysis, bone scans remain a useful supplementary tool in cases where other imaging modalities may be equivocal.

Limitations and Challenges

Bone scans are sensitive to bone pathologies involving increased metabolic activity, but they lack specificity as increased bone activity can be observed in non-pathological conditions as well. Careful correlation with clinical and other imaging findings is essential to avoid misinterpretation.

While bone scans provide valuable functional information about bone metabolism, they lack detailed resolution of anatomic structures. Complementary imaging modalities, such as CT or MRI, are often necessary to precisely define the pathology and its relationship to adjacent structures.

Lastly, it is important to keep in mind that bone scans also involve exposure to ionizing radiation, albeit at a relatively low dose. There should be appropriate clinical suspicion to justify a bone scan for diagnostic or prognostic purposes to minimize unnecessary radiation exposure. Bone scans should not be used for general screening purposes or as first-line imaging.

Future Directions

Hybrid imaging techniques which involve combining bone scans with other imaging modalities, such as SPECT/CT or PET/CT, offer the potential to improve diagnostic accuracy and surgical planning by providing both functional and anatomic information.

Ongoing research into novel radiopharmaceuticals and tracers may also enhance the specificity and sensitivity of bone scans, further improving their diagnostic utility.

Summary

Bone scans serve as valuable tools in spine surgery, providing functional information about bone metabolism and aiding in the diagnosis, surgical planning, and postoperative evaluation of various spinal pathologies. Understanding the strengths and limitations of bone scans is important as bone scans will continue to play an integral role in the evolving landscape of spine surgery.

LOW-DOSE COMPUTED TOMOGRAPHY

CT scans have become a mainstay of spine surgery by providing high-resolution, 3-dimensional images of the bony architecture of the spine and surrounding structures. Traditional CT scans involve substantial radiation exposure, however, raising concerns about potential long-term risks for patients. Low- dose CT scans offer a solution to this challenge, utilizing advanced techniques to maintain diagnostic accuracy while minimizing radiation dose. Low-dose CT scans employ various techniques to reduce radiation exposure. These include lowering tube current, using tube current modulation, and employing iterative reconstruction (IR) algorithms to improve image quality with reduced radiation dose. Low-dose CT scans significantly lower radiation exposure for patients, especially those requiring repeated imaging or vulnerable populations, such as children and pregnant women.

Iterative Reconstruction Techniques

One of the primary methods for reducing radiation in low-dose CT scans is through IR techniques. Traditional CT scans use filtered back projection algorithms, which tend to produce high levels of noise and require higher radiation doses for adequate image quality. On the other hand, IR methods optimize image quality by refining the reconstruction process, resulting in lower noise levels and improved diagnostic information. These techniques enable high-quality images even at reduced radiation levels. Adaptive statistical iterative reduction is a sophisticated algorithm that combines iterative reconstruction with statistical modeling to achieve further reductions in radiation exposure. A study by Alshamari and colleagues showed that IR reduces image noise of low-dose CTs of the lumbar spine in a linear fashion with increased strength of IR compared to conventional filtered back projection.[11] Low-dose CTs with adaptive statistical IR have been shown to lower patient radiation doses by up to 20% while maintaining similar levels of image quality and noise.[13]

Dual-Energy Computed Tomography

Dual-energy CT is an innovative technique that employs 2 different X-ray energy levels during the scan, enabling the differentiation of materials based on their unique energy-dependent properties. This method reduces radiation dose by acquiring 2 datasets at once, which can then be combined to produce detailed images with enhanced tissue contrast and lower noise levels. A recent meta-analysis of dual-energy CT for spine fractures found a sensitivity and specificity of 86.2% and 91.2% for dual-energy CT, which was superior to that of conventional CT at 81.3% and 80.7%, respectively.[15]

Photon Counting Computed Tomography

Photon counting CT is another technology that holds promise in low-dose imaging. Unlike traditional CT, which uses energy-integrating detectors, photon counting CT employs detectors capable of counting individual X-ray photons. This precise detection allows for dose reduction while maintaining image quality. Additionally, photon counting CT offers advanced material decomposition capabilities, making it useful in applications such as bone mineral density assessments and metal artifact reduction. A prospective study of photon counting CT of the spine showed increased sharpness and lower noise levels compared to conventional CT.[16]

Challenges and Considerations

Balancing reduced radiation dose with image quality remains a challenge. Image noise and artifacts may increase with reduced radiation. Surgeons must be cautious when interpreting low-dose CT scans, as image noise and artifacts may affect the visualization of critical structures.

Implementing low-dose CT technology may also require adjustments to current imaging protocols and radiological practices, necessitating training and familiarization for radiologists and technologists. Acquiring and maintaining low-dose CT technology may require significant financial investment and may not be immediately feasible for all health care facilities.

Future Directions

The integration of artificial intelligence and machine learning algorithms may further improve low-dose CT image quality, reducing image noise and artifacts while maintaining diagnostic accuracy. Combining low-dose CT with other imaging modalities such as MRI can also provide comprehensive information while minimizing radiation by as much as possible.

SUMMARY

Low-dose CT scans have emerged as a valuable imaging modality in spine surgery, striking a balance between diagnostic accuracy and minimizing radiation exposure. By implementing novel techniques in image acquisition and processing, low-dose CT scans facilitate diagnoses, preoperative planning, and postsurgical assessments at the lowest radiation dose possible. Surgeons should continue to be mindful of radiation exposure to themselves and their patients and use low-dose CT protocols whenever feasible.

CLINICS CARE POINTS

- Cone-beam CT has proved to be a valuable tool during spine surgery to evaluate accuracy of pedicle screw placement while at the same time being utilized for CT-guided navigation of spinal implants. This has helped decreased the need for reoperations due to misplaced implants. Further refinement of this technology will be focused on decreasing radiation while at the same time improving the imaging detail.

- Synthetic CT has emerged as a valuable tool in spine surgery, providing accurate, radiation-free, 3D imaging of bony anatomy and pathology, while streamlining the preoperative workflow with single-modality imaging. The methods of generating synthetic CT are continuing to be refined, along with its applications in workflow for preoperative planning and intraoperative navigation.

- Low-dose CT scans have emerged as a valuable imaging modality in spine surgery, striking a balance between diagnostic accuracy and minimizing radiation exposure. By implementing novel techniques in image acquisition and processing, low-dose CT scans facilitate diagnoses, preoperative planning, and postsurgical assessments at the lowest radiation dose possible. This has been particularly helpful in certain radiation-sensitive cohorts such as the pediatric population. Surgeons should continue to be mindful of radiation exposure to themselves and their patients and use low-dose CT protocols whenever feasible.

- Bone scans serve as valuable tools in spine surgery, providing functional information about bone metabolism and aiding in the diagnosis, surgical planning, and postoperative evaluation of various spinal pathologies and pseudoarthrosis.

DISCLOSURES

The authors declare no commercial or financial conflicts of interest.

REFERENCES

1. Deyo RA, Gray DT, Kreuter W, et al. United States trends in lumbar fusion surgery for degenerative conditions. Spine (Phila Pa 1976) 2005;30:1441–5.
2. Martin BI, Mirza SK, Spina N, et al. Trends in Lumbar Fusion Procedure Rates and Associated Hospital Costs for Degenerative Spinal Diseases in the United States, 2004 to 2015. Spine (Phila Pa 1976) 2019;44:369–76.
3. Hagan MJ, Syed S, Leary OP, et al. Pedicle Screw Placement Using Intraoperative Computed Tomography and Computer-Aided Spinal Navigation Improves Screw Accuracy and Avoids Postoperative Revisions: Single-Center Analysis of 1400 Pedicle Screws. World Neurosurg 2022;160:e169–79.
4. Farah K, Coudert P, Graillon T, et al. Prospective Comparative Study in Spine Surgery Between O-Arm and Airo Systems: Efficacy and Radiation Exposure. World Neurosurg 2018;118:e175–84.
5. Ille S, Baumgart L, Obermueller T, et al. Clinical efficiency of operating room-based sliding gantry CT as compared to mobile cone-beam CT-based navigated pedicle screw placement in 853 patients and 6733 screws. Eur Spine J 2021;30:3720–30.
6. Lenski M, Hofereiter J, Terpolilli N, et al. Dual-room CT with a sliding gantry for intraoperative imaging: feasibility and workflow analysis of an interdisciplinary concept. Int J Comput Assist Radiol Surg 2019;14:397–407.
7. Laine T, Lund T, Ylikoski M, et al. Accuracy of pedicle screw insertion with and without computer assistance: A randomised controlled clinical study in 100 consecutive patients. Eur Spine J 2000;9:235–40.
8. Hecht N, Yassin H, Czabanka M, et al. Intraoperative Computed Tomography Versus 3D C-Arm Imaging for Navigated Spinal Instrumentation. Spine (Phila Pa 1976) 2018;43:370–7.
9. Malham GM, Wells-Quinn T. What should my hospital buy next?—Guidelines for the acquisition and application of imaging, navigation, and robotics for spine surgery. Journal of Spine Surgery 2019. https://doi.org/10.21037/jss.2019.02.04.
10. Gelalis ID, Paschos NK, Pakos EE, et al. Accuracy of pedicle screw placement: A systematic review of prospective in vivo studies comparing free hand, fluoroscopy guidance and navigation techniques. Eur Spine J 2012. https://doi.org/10.1007/s00586-011-2011-3.
11. Alshamari M, Geijer M, Norrman E, et al. Impact of iterative reconstruction on image quality of low-dose CT of the lumbar spine. Acta Radiol 2017;58:702–9.
12. Fichtner J, et al. Revision Rate of Misplaced Pedicle Screws of the Thoracolumbar Spine–Comparison of Three-Dimensional Fluoroscopy Navigation with Freehand Placement: A Systematic Analysis and Review of the Literature. World Neurosurg 2018;109:e24–32.
13. Komlosi P, et al. Adaptive statistical iterative reconstruction reduces patient radiation dose in neuroradiology CT studies. Neuroradiology 2014;56:187–93.
14. Amrhein TJ, Schauberger JS, Kranz PG, et al. Reducing patient radiation exposure from CT fluoroscopy-guided lumbar spine pain injections by targeting the planning CT. Am J Roentgenol 2016;206:390–4.
15. Bäcker HC, Wu CH, Perka C, et al. Dual-energy computed tomography in spine fractures: A systematic review and meta-analysis. Internet J Spine Surg 2021;15:525–35.
16. Rau A, et al. Photon-Counting Computed Tomography (PC-CT) of the spine: impact on diagnostic confidence and radiation dose. Eur Radiol 2023;33.

17. Yson SC, et al. Comparison of cranial facet joint violation rates between open and percutaneous pedicle screw placement using intraoperative 3-D CT (o-arm) computer navigation. Spine (Phila Pa 1976) 2013;38.

18. Shin BJ, James AR, Njoku IU, et al. Pedicle screw navigation: A systematic review and meta-analysis of perforation risk for computer-navigated versus freehand insertion - A review. J Neurosurg Spine 2012. https://doi.org/10.3171/2012.5.SPINE11399.

19. Ughwanogho E, Patel NM, Baldwin KD, et al. Computed tomography-guided navigation of thoracic pedicle screws for adolescent idiopathic scoliosis results in more accurate placement and less screw removal. Spine (Phila Pa 1976) 2012;37.

20. Schouten R, Lee R, Boyd M, et al. Intra-operative cone-beam CT (O-arm) and stereotactic navigation in acute spinal trauma surgery. J Clin Neurosci 2012;19:1137–43.

21. Kumar M, Shanavas M, Sidappa A, et al. Cone beam computed tomography - know its secrets. J Int Oral Health 2015;7:64–8.

22. Efird JT, Jindal C, Podder TK, et al. Cone beam computed tomography-the need for future guidance. J Thorac Dis 2022. https://doi.org/10.21037/jtd-22-1008.

23. National Council on Radiation Protection and Measurements. 45. National Council on Radiation Protection and Measurements. Radiation protection in dentistry.

24. Rousseau J, Dreuil S, Bassinet C, et al. Surgivisio® and O-arm®O2 cone beam CT mobile systems for guidance of lumbar spine surgery: Comparison of patient radiation dose. Phys Med 2021;85:192–9.

25. Casiraghi M, Scarone P, Bellesi L, et al. Effective dose and image quality for intraoperative imaging with a cone-beam CT and a mobile multi-slice CT in spinal surgery: A phantom study. Phys Med 2021;81:9–19.

26. Winn N, Kaur S, Cassar-Pullicino V, et al. A novel use of cone beam CT: flexion and extension weight-bearing imaging to assess spinal stability. Eur Spine J 2022;31:1667–81.

27. Härtl R, Lam KS, Wang J, et al. Worldwide survey on the use of navigation in spine surgery. World Neurosurgery 2013;79 162–172. https://doi.org/10.1016/j.wneu.2012.03.011. Preprint at.

28. Staartjes VE, Seevinck PR, Vandertop WP, et al. Magnetic resonance imaging–based synthetic computed tomography of the lumbar spine for surgical planning: a clinical proof-of-concept. Neurosurg Focus 2021;50:1–7.

29. Bohl DD, Hijji FY, Massel DH, et al. Patient knowledge regarding radiation exposure from spinal imaging. Spine J 2017;17:305–12.

30. Biswas D, Bible JE, Bohan M, et al. Radiation exposure from musculoskeletal computerized tomographic scans. J Bone Joint Surg 2009;91:1882–9.

31. Lin EC. Radiation risk from medical imaging. Mayo Clin Proc 2010;85:1142–6.

32. Papachristodoulou, A. et al. Radiation dose of lumbar spine CT: analysis and comparison between different modes of acquisition in two European imaging centers. www.myESR.org.

33. Richards PJ, George J, Metelko M, et al. Spine computed tomography doses and cancer induction. Spine (Phila Pa 1976) 2010;35:430–3.

34. Upadhyay J, Iwasaka-Neder J, Golden E, et al. Synthetic CT Assessment of Lesions in Children With Rare Musculoskeletal Diseases. Pediatrics 2023;152.

35. Boulanger M, Nunes JC, Chourak H, et al. Deep learning methods to generate synthetic CT from MRI in radiotherapy: A literature review. Phys Med 2021. https://doi.org/10.1016/j.ejmp.2021.07.027.

36. Lee JH, Han IH, Kim DH, et al. Spine computed tomography to magnetic resonance image synthesis using generative adversarial networks: A preliminary study. J Korean Neurosurg Soc 2020;63:386–96.

37. Gersing AS, Pfeiffer D, Kopp FK, et al. Evaluation of MR-derived CT-like images and simulated radiographs compared to conventional radiography in patients with benign and malignant bone tumors. Eur Radiol 2019;29:13–21.

38. Argentieri EC, Koff MF, Breighner RE, et al. Diagnostic Accuracy of Zero-Echo Time MRI for the Evaluation of Cervical Neural Foraminal Stenosis. Spine (Phila Pa 1976) 2018;43:928–33.

39. Breighner RE, Bogner EA, Lee SC, et al. Evaluation of Osseous Morphology of the Hip Using Zero Echo Time Magnetic Resonance Imaging. Am J Sports Med 2019;47:3460–8.

40. Florkow MC, Zijlstra F, Willemsen K, et al. Deep learning–based MR-to-CT synthesis: The influence of varying gradient echo–based MR images as input channels. Magn Reson Med 2020;83:1429–41.

41. van der Kolk B, Britt) YM, et al. Bone visualization of the cervical spine with deep learning-based synthetic CT compared to conventional CT: A single-center noninferiority study on image quality. Eur J Radiol 2022;154.

42. Morbée L, et al. MRI-based synthetic CT of the hip: can it be an alternative to conventional CT in the evaluation of osseous morphology? Eur Radiol 2022;32:3112–20.

43. Roberts M, Hinton G, Wells AJ, et al. Imaging evaluation of a proposed 3D generative model for MRI to CT translation in the lumbar spine. Spine J 2023. https://doi.org/10.1016/j.spinee.2023.06.399.

44. Jeong HS, Park C, Kim KS, et al. Clinical feasibility of MR-generated synthetic CT images of the cervical spine: Diagnostic performance for detection of OPLL and comparison of CT number. Medicine (United States) 2021;100:E25800.

45. Al-Riyami K, Gnanasegaran G, Van den Wyngaert T, et al. Bone SPECT/CT in the postoperative spine: a focus on spinal fusion. Eur J Nucl Med Mol Imag 2017. https://doi.org/10.1007/s00259-017-3765-6.

46. van Stralen M, Podlogar M, Hendrikse J, et al. BoneMRI of the cervical spine: Deep learning-based radiodensity contrast generation for selective visualization of osseous structures. ISMRM 27th Annual Meeting and Exhibition. May 11-16, 2019. Available at: https://archive.ismrm.org/2019/1142.html.

47. Edmund JM, Nyholm T. A review of substitute CT generation for MRI-only radiation therapy. Radiat Oncol 2017. https://doi.org/10.1186/s13014-016-0747-y.

48. Hofmann M, Pichler B, Schölkopf B, et al. Towards quantitative PET/MRI: A review of MR-based attenuation correction techniques. Eur J Nucl Med Mol Imaging 2009;36:93–104.

49. Baldwin LN, Wachowicz K, Thomas SD, et al. Characterization, prediction, and correction of geometric distortion in 3 T MR images. Med Phys 2007;34: 388–99.

50. Love C, Palestro CJ. Nuclear medicine imaging of bone infections. Clin Radiol 2016;71:632–46.

51. Gates GF, McDonald RJ. Bone SPECT of the back after lumbar surgery. Clin Nucl Med 1999;24: 395–403.

52. Nouh MR. Spinal fusion-hardware construct: Basic concepts and imaging review. World J Radiol 2012;4:193.

53. Gruskay JA, Webb ML, Grauer JN. Methods of evaluating lumbar and cervical fusion. Spine J 2014. https://doi.org/10.1016/j.spinee.2013.07.459.

54. Heimburger C, et al. Bone scan SPECT/CT for the diagnosis of late complications after spinal fusion: Definition and evaluation of interpretation criteria. Med Nucl 2015;39:105–21.

55. Hudyana H, Maes A, Vandenberghe T, et al. Accuracy of bone SPECT/CT for identifying hardware loosening in patients who underwent lumbar fusion with pedicle screws. Eur J Nucl Med Mol Imaging 2016;43:349–54.

56. Ledonio CGT, Burton DC, Crawford CH, et al. Current Evidence Regarding Diagnostic Imaging Methods for Pediatric Lumbar Spondylolysis: A Report From the Scoliosis Research Society Evidence-Based Medicine Committee. Spine Deform 2017;5:97–101.

Image-Guided Spine Surgery

Khanathip Jitpakdee, MD[a], Blake Boadi, BS[b], Roger Härtl, MD[b],*

KEYWORDS

- Image-guided spine surgery • Spine surgery • Imaging • Navigation • Technology
- Computed tomography • Minimally invasive spine surgery

KEY POINTS

- Image guidance and navigation in spine surgery combine preoperative or intraoperative imaging data with precise location tracking system of the surgical instrument.
- This technology provides comprehensive view of surgical anatomy, allowing surgeons to perform surgery with greater precision while reducing radiation exposure.
- Different types of imaging technology and navigation systems are available, including intraoperative and preoperative image acquisition, 2D and 3D reconstruction images, optical and electromagnetic navigation, etc.
- Image-guided navigation serves as a foundation for incorporating other advanced technologies like augmented reality and robotics into spine surgery.

INTRODUCTION

Rapid technological advancements have significantly impacted spine surgery and spinal instrumentation through the continuous development of complex surgical techniques and well-developed spinal implants. With the progression of knowledge and surgical techniques, spine surgery has become increasingly complicated and challenging, especially with the introduction of minimally invasive spine surgery (MISS). MISS has become popular as one of the standard treatments for spinal disorders with proven advantages over traditional open surgery. However, with a minimally invasive approach, direct visualization of anatomic landmarks is compromised by the limited surgical visual field. This underscores the importance of minimizing potential complications such as dural tears, spinal cord or nerve root injury, vascular injuries, or iatrogenic instability from violation of stabilizing structures. Achieving this goal necessitates the surgeon's experience and a thorough understanding of surgical anatomy, which can be greatly facilitated by intraoperative imaging. Therefore, reliance on imaging technology becomes crucial to help surgeons precisely recognize the anatomic structures as well as the position of spinal instruments. This imaging technology allows precise orientation even when anatomic structures shift during surgery or when the surgical field is limited, particularly in MISS.

The rising trend of MISS has led to reliance on image guidance, particularly intraoperative fluoroscopy at the beginning of development stages. This preference stems from the fact that minimal muscle dissection and operation through a small exposure inside a tubular retractor in MISS usually hinders proper visualization of the anatomic landmarks, as opposed to traditional open surgery where the surgical anatomy is extensively exposed and collateral injury to the surrounding structure is inevitable. While 3-dimensional (3D) navigation enhances instrument precision and minimizes radiation exposure, its adoption in clinical practice faces obstacles due to its associated costs and surgeon's concerns of potential prolonged

[a] Department of Orthopedics, Queen Savang Vadhana Memorial Hospital, Thai Red Cross Society, 290 Jermjompol, Si Racha, Chonburi 20110, Thailand; [b] Department of Neurosurgery, Weill Cornell Medicine, New York-Presbyterian - Och Spine, 525 East 68th Street, Box 99, New York, NY 10021, USA
* Corresponding author.
E-mail address: roh9005@med.cornell.edu

Neurosurg Clin N Am 35 (2024) 173–190
https://doi.org/10.1016/j.nec.2023.11.008
1042-3680/24/© 2023 Elsevier Inc. All rights reserved.

operative times, usability, seamless integration into surgical workflows, and safety considerations. To address these concerns, it is essential to focus on the advancement of imaging technologies, the improvement of image quality, and the accuracy of navigation systems. Additionally, practicing through a step-by-step workflow that involves both the surgeon and the operative room staff is crucial for overcoming these challenges and achieving proficiency in intraoperative image-guided navigation. This approach facilitates a smoother learning curve and improves the effectiveness and safety of the procedure.

Our institutions have integrated image-guided technologies to aid in a wide range of spinal surgery procedures, with a particular focus on MISS for various conditions like degenerative diseases, deformity correction, trauma, and spinal tumors. By utilizing different navigational systems over time, we have experienced the evolution from traditional fluoroscopy to advanced techniques such as 3D fluoroscopic navigation, preoperative, intraoperative 3D computed tomography (CT) navigation, augmented reality-assisted spine surgery, and spinal robotics. This chapter presents an overview of types of image acquisition, tracking systems, registration systems, along with their benefits and limitations. Additionally, the surgical workflows for image-guided spine surgery are illustrated, shedding light on the current practices in this field. We also introduced the concept of "Total Navigation" through the integration of intraoperative 3D CT navigation that we regularly use in every surgical step of spine surgery. Finally, the chapter touches upon the potential future advancements and applications of image-guided systems within spine surgery.

HISTORICAL ADVANCEMENT OF IMAGE-GUIDED SPINE SURGERY

The development of this imaging technology has been a lengthy process, spanning numerous years. The journey of medical imaging began with the discovery of X-rays back in 1895 by Wilhelm Roentgen. Subsequent breakthroughs, such as the development of X-ray image intensifiers in the 1940s which allowed for captures of the fluoroscopic images by the C-arm in 1955 and advancements in computational science, paved the way for a remarkable innovation known as computed tomography which was introduced by Godfrey Hounsfield in 1971. During the late 1980s, there were notable advancements in stereotactic imaging, and in 1998, the introduction of 4-row detector CT scanners brought about a significant breakthrough in 3D reconstruction

capabilities.[1] This pivotal imaging technology played a crucial role in propelling the rapid evolution of modern navigational technologies that we use today since these advancements led to a remarkable transformation in neuronavigational systems. In 2004, the world saw the introduction of robotics in spine surgery, a significant leap in medical technology. This integration of cutting-edge technologies made it possible to achieve safer procedures and consistently accurate placements of pedicle screws. Today, robotics in spine surgery has become a reliable and effective modality, revolutionizing the field, and improving patient outcomes. Historical advancements related to the image-guided spine surgery and navigation are illustrated in the timeline in **Fig. 1**.

NON-NAVIGATED 2-DIMENSIONAL FLUOROSCOPY

Currently, C-arm fluoroscopy is 1 of the most common intraoperative imaging modalities used in spine surgery, especially for percutaneous pedicle screw insertion (**Fig. 2**). Fluoroscopy offers precise localization of the target area, relatively low initial investment in equipment, quick setup, easy learning curve, and versatility across different procedures within the hospital setting. However, it comes with some drawbacks. The radiation exposure is unavoidable, particularly concerning in complex surgeries where higher radiation dosages may be needed. Moreover, fluoroscopy provides 2-dimensional (2D) images which require obtaining images from multiple planes, and lack continuous, real-time information on the surgical instrument's position, leading to challenges in interpretation. This limitation becomes particularly problematic in operations involving severe spinal deformities, making it difficult to obtain true anteroposterior and lateral fluoroscopic views. This can increase the risk of misplaced pedicle screws or instrumentation. Furthermore, surgeons typically need to temporarily pause the operation and introduce the fluoroscope to acquire intraoperative images before they can continue the surgical workflow. In response to these shortcomings, innovative intraoperative image-guided navigation techniques have been developed to overcome these challenges.

CLASSIFICATION OF IMAGE-GUIDED NAVIGATION IN SPINE SURGERY

Various methods exist to categorize imaging modalities for spine surgery, and these classifications can be based on factors such as the timing of image acquisition, image quality, or the type of tracking systems employed (**Fig. 3**).

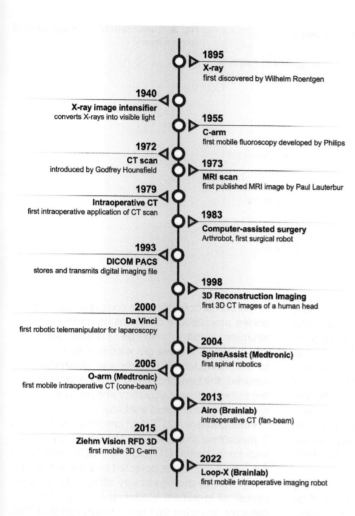

Timing of Image Acquisition: Preoperative and Intraoperative Imaging

Images that are used for spinal navigation can be acquired preoperatively or intraoperatively.

Preoperative images can be obtained from thin-cut CT scans prior to surgery to create a virtual 3D reconstruction using a navigational workstation. This reconstruction serves as a valuable tool for surgical planning, aiding in the determination

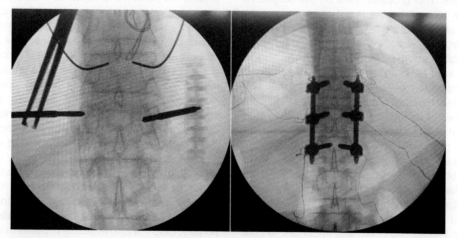

Fig. 2. Fluoroscopic non-navigated 2D images obtained to assist percutaneous pedicle screw insertion for thoracolumbar burst fracture.

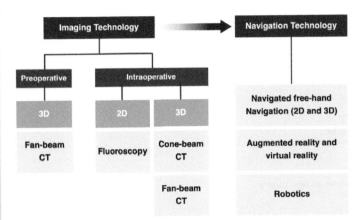

Fig. 3. Classifications of image-guided spine surgery.

of the ideal trajectory for pedicle screw insertion, appropriate screw dimensions, and even simulating other implants like connecting rods or interbody cages. However, it is important to note that preoperative CT scans are typically acquired while the patient is in a supine position, whereas the spine surgery is typically performed with the patient in a prone position. This difference in position can result in changes of spinal alignment and vertebral position mismatch, potentially leading to navigation errors and complications from inaccuracy.

To address this issue and ensure accuracy during surgery, each level of the spine must be registered separately, accounting for the changing alignment. This registration process involves selecting specific anatomic landmarks on the preoperative CT images and correlating them with the patient's intraoperative anatomy. However, CT-based guidance systems have certain drawbacks. This process relies on the surgeon's expertise to perform the registration accurately, which can introduce a degree of variability. Moreover, achieving accurate registration often necessitates additional bony exposure, and in patients who have undergone prior decompressive laminectomy, identifying landmarks for registration can be challenging. These factors should be taken into consideration when using preoperative CT-based navigation systems for spine surgery.

During surgery, 2D or 3D intraoperative images can be obtained using fluoroscopy or CT, eliminating the issues related to positional changes and realignment. This ensures that the navigation is based on the most current and accurate anatomic images. However, it is important to note that acquiring these intraoperative images will add

to the overall operative time compared to using imported preoperative CT scans. In addition, the instrument position can be planned after the intraoperative images are successfully transferred to the workstation. Despite the additional time required, the benefit of using intraoperative images lies in the improved accuracy and up-to-date visualization of the surgical anatomy.

Intraoperative 3D CT data can be acquired using 2 modalities: conventional fan beam CT (FBCT) and cone beam CT (CBCT). FBCT employs a fan-type X-ray that is detected by a linear detector array. The system geometry effectively prevents almost all in-patient scattering from reaching the detector, ensuring that only primary radiation that passed through the patient reaches the detector and contributes to the reconstructed data. On the other hand, CBCT is a more recent imaging modality that utilizes a cone-type X-ray. This emission is detected by a flat panel sensor that rotates around the patient and captures imaging data in a cone-shaped X-ray beam, while FBCT captures images as slices. Projection images in multiple planes are generated by the X-ray source and detector array which rotate 180 to 360° around the patient. These images are then reconstructed using computer algorithms to produce high-resolution 3D images. FBCT provides superior soft tissue definition and bone resolution compared to CBCT. The images obtained from a fan-type X-ray exhibit greater spatial and contrast resolution, whereas CBCT is affected by a higher amount of scatter radiation occurring within the larger beam. CBCT offers advantages such as lower radiation dosage, reduced cost, and fewer artifacts when dealing with metallic objects. Additionally, CBCT is also available in the form of a mobile 3D C-arm system (3D fluoroscopy), providing a more compact and comfortable option for intraoperative use (**Fig. 4**A-C).

Types of Acquired Image Quality: 2-Dimensional and 3-Dimensional Navigation

The 2D navigation technique involves the integration of computer-assisted guidance into the surgical process to work with conventional fluoroscopic images. A tracker is attached to the patient, and fluoroscopic anteroposterior and lateral images are obtained. A fixed reference frame is applied to the surgical field, and the instruments used in the surgery are equipped with tags to track their positions in relation to the surgical field. Once intraoperative fluoroscopic images are obtained and imported to the workstation, the surgical instruments fitted with light-emitting diodes are detected by a camera. Subsequently, these instrument positions are virtually projected onto the fluoroscopy monitor on 2D fluoroscopic images as backgrounds (**Fig. 5**). This advanced approach significantly enhances precision and visualization during the surgical procedure. The utilization of this approach offers several benefits, including its speed, reduced radiation exposure for both the surgeon and the patient, and its simplicity. However, it is not without limitations. The primary drawback lies in its reliance on a 2D virtual navigation system, making it more prone to errors and

misinterpretations when compared to a comprehensive 3D rendering. Moreover, the image quality can be diminished by similar factors that compromise fluoroscopic image quality, such as thick soft tissue shadow in obese patients, shoulder and scapular shadow in lower cervical and thoracic spine, or interference from radio-opaque materials. As a result, the next generation of more advanced 3D-guided navigation systems has been shown to offer superior accuracy, overcoming these shortcomings and enhancing the precision of surgical procedures.[2]

On the other hand, 3D-CT navigation presents a distinct contrast, offering greater clarity in visualizing the spinal anatomy in axial, coronal, and sagittal planes. This navigation technique also involves securely affixing a registration tracker to the patient's body, which is then combined with images from preoperative or intraoperative CT images or 3D fluoroscopy. During the registration process, bony landmarks within the CT scan and the patient's anatomy are identified, and a transformation matrix is calculated to complete the registration. Navigation cameras track the reflected infrared light from reflective spheres (light-emitting diodes) which are attached to surgical instruments. Consequently, the surgeon gains the ability to navigate the patient's spinal anatomy through a visual representation that displays the position of the tracked instruments superimposed

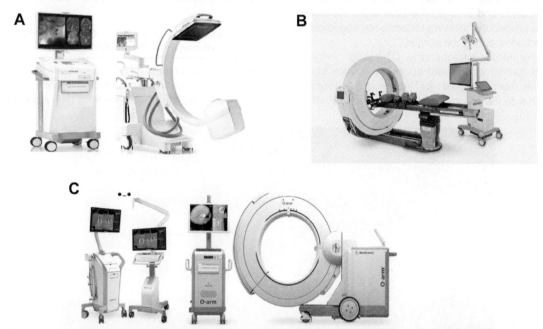

Fig. 4. Intraoperative image-guided navigation system (*A*) 3D fluoroscopy (Ziehm Vision RFD 3D®. With permission from © 2023 Ziehm Imaging GmbH.), (*B*) 3D fan beam computed tomography (Airo TruCT®. With permission from © Stryker.), and (*C*) 3D cone beam computed tomography (O-Arm®. Images from Medtronic, plc © 2024.). In 2013 Airo was created by Mobius. Airo was only sold by the Brainlab sales team, Then Stryker acquired Airo in 2019.

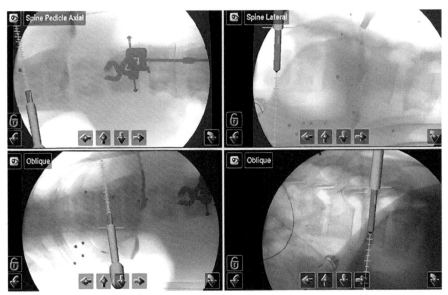

Fig. 5. 2D fluoroscopic image-guided percutaneous pedicle screw insertion.[3]

in the 3D CT images, allowing a more precise and comprehensive understanding during the surgical procedure. During percutaneous pedicle screw insertion, the selected screw entry point and trajectory are superimposed on these images. As adjustments are made to the chosen trajectory within the surgical field, this visual information is continually updated in real-time (**Fig. 6**). This dynamic feedback loop empowers the surgeon with precise guidance and a comprehensive understanding of the procedure, allowing for accurate and informed decisions during the surgery.

For MISS, intraoperative CT-based navigation has gained widespread adoption. Several studies have demonstrated its ability to significantly enhance the accuracy of pedicle screw placement,

reduce facet violation, and minimize radiation exposure when compared to fluoroscopy-based navigation. The focus on achieving the utmost precision in real time renders CT navigation exceptionally well-suited for implementation in minimally invasive approaches, where precise localization plays a critical role in achieving successful outcomes. Comparison of common types of intraoperative spinal navigation is depicted in **Table 1**.

Navigation Tracking Systems: Optical-Based and Electromagnetic-Based Navigation

There are 2 main types of tracking systems used in spinal surgery: optical and electromagnetic systems. Currently, the optical tracking navigation is

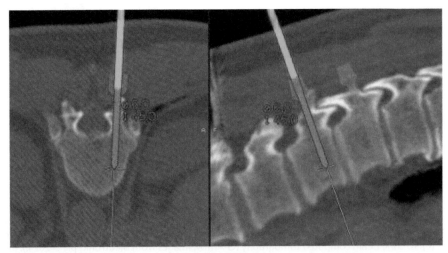

Fig. 6. 3D CT image-guided percutaneous pedicle screw insertion.

Table 1
Comparison of different types of common spinal navigation[4–7]

	Navigated 2D Fluoroscopy	Preoperative 3D CT	Intraoperative 3D Cone Beam CT	Intraoperative 3D Fan Beam CT
Type of acquired image	2D (AP and lateral X-ray)	3D	3D	3D
Intraoperative image acquisition	Needed	No needed	Needed	Needed
Actual real time image	Possible if needed	No	Possible if needed	Possible if needed
Image resolution and quality	Low	Excellent	Moderate	Excellent
Soft tissue image quality	Not available	Good	Poor	Good
Average scanning time	< 30 s	30 s	30–45 s	30 s
Duration of registration	Short	Long	Short	Very short
Field of view	Limited (3–5 vertebra)	Widest (Whole spine)	Wide (6–8 vertebra)	Widest (Whole spine)
Use in severe spinal deformity	Not suitable	Good	Possible	Good
Radiation dose delivered Patient	Low	High	Moderate	High
Surgeon	Low	None	Low	Low
Simplicity of use	Good	Moderate	Moderate	More advanced
Specialized operating table	Not required	Not required	Not required	Required
Added operative time	Moderate	Low	High	High
Accuracy	Good	High	High	Highest
Cost	Low	Moderate	High	High

Abbreviations: 2D, 2-dimensional; 3D, 3-dimensional; CT, computed tomography.

the more commonly integrated system in spinal surgeries. These systems rely on infrared cameras for tracking the light emitted or reflected from the attached light-emitting diodes (LEDs) or reflective spheres on the reference array and navigational instruments. This real-time tracking provides real-time location of the handheld surgical instruments in relation to the anatomy in the surgical field. Utilizing infrared wavelengths helps reduce distortion that could potentially arise from any nearby metal or electrical fields within the operating room. However, it is essential to maintain a continuous "line of sight" between the LEDs, the navigation instruments, and the specialized cameras throughout the procedure because any objects obstructing this line of sight, including surgeon's movement, blood stains or small tissue debris on the reflective spheres, can interfere with the infrared tracking process. Furthermore, to keep the navigation accuracy during the procedure, the stability of the reference array and the distance between the LEDs and relevant surgical anatomy must remain unchanged compared to the initial registration.

The issue of line-of-sight limitations can sometimes restrict the surgeon's natural range of movement, impeding handling of instruments and potentially causing discomfort in ergonomics during surgery. In contrast, electromagnetic navigation systems have been developed to overcome these limitations (**Fig. 7**A and B). These systems operate based on a specialized field generator positioned near the surgical field, which creates an electromagnetic field, along with a patient tracker and a signal coil for surgical instruments. To register the patient's surgical anatomy, a patient tracker is securely attached to the anatomic reference point such as the ilium or spinous process. The surgical instruments are equipped with sensor

A   **B**

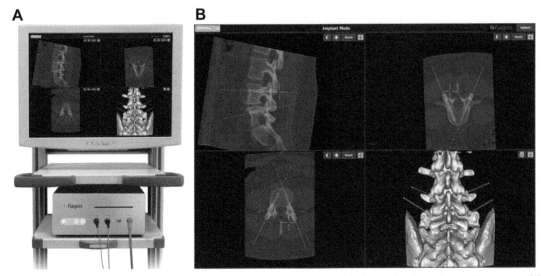

Fig. 7. Electromagnetic-based navigation for pedicle screw insertion (*A*) Control unit with monitor screen (*B*) Navigated images for screw entry point, size, and trajectory. ([A,B] With permission from© 2022 Fiagon GmbH.)

signal coils, allowing the electromagnetic navigation system to determine their positions in relation to the registered spinal column. Real-time tracking of instrument positions is achieved by detecting their relationship to the patient's anatomy through sensing changes in the electromagnetic field produced by the field generator. Unlike optical navigation, electromagnetic tracking systems are not affected by line-of-sight interference, allowing for a continuous signaling in the electromagnetic field.[7] Furthermore, electromagnetic navigation offers the advantage of being more lightweight and comfortable to handle, compared to optical-based systems where the inclusion of reflective LEDs adds to the size and weight of the instruments. Nevertheless, it is crucial to note that significant interference and field distortion leading to deviated accuracies may arise in the navigational images due to metal artifacts and electromagnetic fields emanating from other frequently used operating room devices in proximity to the electromagnetic field, such as cardiac pacemakers, cochlear implants, electrocautery, and electrocardiogram monitoring equipment.[8–10] (**Table 2**)

REGISTRATION SYSTEMS
Manual Registration: Paired-Point Matching and Surface Matching

Manual registration involves matching multiple anatomic points from a preoperative or intraoperative data to the patient's position on the operating table. Typically, these points are planned and acquired based on surgically accessible anatomic landmarks. While manual registration is a quick process, it does involve a few more active steps by the surgeon. To use manual registration, a visible and accessible

bony surface on the exposed posterior element, such as the spinous process or vertebral laminae, is required. By mapping the positional information of the posterior surface of a vertebra with a pointer, the navigation system creates a topographic map, matching the orientation and anatomic position with the acquired image (**Fig. 8**). One of the benefits from manual registration is the potential to reduce radiation exposure to the patient and the surgical team, as fewer scans may be needed. This method is also useful for re-registration when the patient reference is accidently moved, often without the need for additional scans. However, a potential disadvantage of this technique is the risk of navigational inaccuracy if the surgeon makes errors in selecting specific anatomic points in the surgical field. Combining the paired-point and surface matching approaches has been shown to result in significantly higher accuracy during the navigation process.[16]

CT-fluoro matching is an alternative registration method employed when the navigation system is based on preoperative CT images. With this technique, the preoperative CT scan is aligned with intraoperative 2D fluoroscopic images of the patient's spine, captured from various angles. By utilizing CT-fluoro matching navigation, surgeons benefit from improved intraoperative visualization of bony structures and improved precision in screw placement, all while minimizing radiation exposure.[17]

Automatic Registration

Automatic image registration becomes feasible in the presence of a reference array or markers on the intraoperative scanner, including a fluoroscope or CT. The patient is equipped with another

Table 2
Comparison of optical- and electromagnetic-based navigation[7,11–15]

	Optical-based Navigation	EM-Based Navigation
Navigation system component	Infrared tracking camera, light-emitting diodes, and reference array	Electromagnetic field generator, patient tracker, and signal coils
Mode of registration	Surface matching, paired-point, automated registration	Surface registration
Registration time	Slightly longer	Slightly shorter
Accuracy	Very high	Comparable (further studies required)
Rigid immobilization of the surgical area	Needed	Not required
Added weight to surgical instrument	Added weight from attached reflective spheres	Lightweight
Convenience in instrument handling	Free handling (wireless) but need to maintain line-of-sight	Wired instrument
Line-of-sight occlusion	Yes	No
Signal interruption from ferromagnetic materials	No	Yes
Occupying space of the system component	Large camera and reference array	Compact EM generator box and patient tracker
Intraoperative radiation exposure Patient Surgeon/staffs	Increase Decrease	None None
Stage of technological advancement	Developing stage with widespread use	Early stage of implementation and adoption
Cost-effectiveness	Economically justified	Further studies required

Abbreviations: EM, electromagnetic.

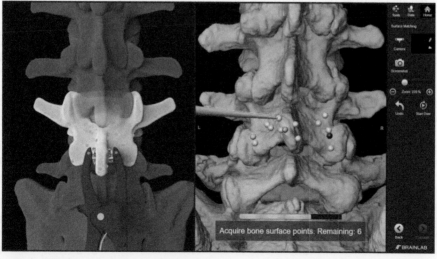

Fig. 8. Manual registration by surface matching—multiple anatomic points on posterior bone surface are selected to match the image dataset. (With permission from © 2023 Brainlab AG.)

reference array, allowing the anatomic position to be identified during scanning. This registration process is only possible when the image acquisition is performed intraoperatively. The acquired images are then automatically transferred to the navigation system, where patient registration is accomplished. A verification step is included to allow the surgeon to confirm the registration. Automated registration operates independently, eliminating the need for surgeon input and reducing the potential for registration errors. This registration process is particularly beneficial as it enables faster and more comfortable workflow with minimal additional effort.

How image-guided navigation amplifies spinal surgery

Accuracy The incorporation of image-guided navigation has brought significant advancements in the precision and efficiency of spinal procedures, particularly in MISS. In situations where the visual field is limited, such as with a small tubular retractor, identifying accurate anatomic landmarks can be challenging. Therefore, the implementation of precise navigation becomes vital to ensure accurate surgical trajectory, as even minor misdirection can lead to prolonged operation times and potential harm to critical structures. Compared to traditional freehand pedicle screw placement, navigation-assisted positioning of pedicle screws has shown significantly reduced misplacement rates. Published studies have analyzed pedicle placements and reported an impressive accuracy rate of more than 96% when utilizing intraoperative CT-based navigation.[18,19] Intraoperative navigation, particularly for percutaneous procedure, aids in determining the optimal entry point from the skin to the pedicle. The implementation of navigation has significantly reduced pedicle perforation rates to lower than 5%. The accuracy of intraoperative 3D CT navigation is shown to be superior to 2D navigation or virtual fluoroscopy.[20,21] During spinal decompression procedures, surgeons can benefit from real-time 3D anatomy localization, allowing for precise identification of the neural foramen and essential stabilizing structures like facet joints. This capability helps surgeons overcome the challenges of a narrow field of view, to achieve adequate bony decompression while avoiding potential complications such as dural tears, vascular injuries, and unnecessary excessive facet joint resection which could lead to postoperative instability. Research findings indicate that 3D CT navigation helps achieve precise pedicle screw trajectory with optimal screw length, size, and angulation, leading to increased pull-out strength compared to non-navigated fluoroscopic guidance. Additionally, the use of intraoperative 3D CT navigation is associated with a lower rate of adjacent facet joint violation from pedicle screw placement.[22,23]

Spinal navigation also benefits in mitigating the risk of wrong-level operations. Interpreting fluoroscopic images in the cervical spine or thoracic spine can be challenging due to radiographic shadowing from body parts like the shoulder girdle and upper chest, which may obscure the spine. Moreover, significant soft tissue in obese patients further complicates the visualization during surgery.[24] Navigation also has a role in spinal tumor operation. Our center has reported a series of microscopic tubular resection of intradural extramedullary tumors with successful results. These procedures were performed using intraoperative navigation to localize the tumor boundaries and resections were done with minimally invasive tubular retractors and the operative microscope.[25]

In such cases, the precision and real-time guidance provided by navigation systems become beneficial for accurate and successful procedures.

Radiation safety For spine surgeons, intraoperative imaging guidance is essential regardless of the type of operation. While it is necessary, the use of intraoperative imaging raises concerns about increasing radiation dosage, which affects both patients and operative team. In MISS, surgeons have to access pathologies through percutaneous incisions or work in small tubular retractors, making it challenging to identify the proper surgical trajectory and anatomic landmarks for pedicle screw placement. Consequently, non-navigated 2D fluoroscopy is used throughout the procedure, resulting in significant radiation exposure. One of the advantages of intraoperative navigation is its ability to significantly reduce radiation exposure for both the surgeon and medical staff, as they are protected during the scanning procedure. After completing image acquisition, either optical or electromagnetic navigation eliminate the risk of radiation exposure during surgery. Intraoperative CT has been shown to reduce radiation exposure time for MISS by over 80% compared to fluoroscopy.[26] However, patients are required to remain in the radiation field during intraoperative image acquisition, potentially resulting in a relatively high dose of radiation exposure when obtaining 3D fluoroscopy or CT images.

Learning curve Navigation technology has been shown to shorten the learning curve for spine surgery. As mentioned earlier, performing MISS can be particularly challenging for novice surgeons, as it demands precise entry points and accurate surgical trajectories. With conventional 2D non-navigated fluoroscopy, surgeons must possess a comprehensive understanding of anatomy, interpret 2D images proficiently, and have adequate experience to achieve efficacy and safety during MISS. However, spinal navigation addresses this issue and facilitates safer training in surgical education. Prior studies have demonstrated that integrating navigation significantly improves trainees' accuracy, reduces operative time, and lowers the revision rate for pedicle screw placements, bringing their performance to a level similar to that of experienced surgeons.[27] Navigation also proves beneficial in endoscopic spine surgery, especially in challenging transforaminal approaches for beginners. Intraoperative 3D navigation enables surgeons to accurately target the neural foramen with less radiation exposure without causing damage to the nerve root. These results highlight how navigation can rapidly improve skills in screw placement and a minimally invasive approach and reduce the technical complexities of spine surgery, as compared to a trial-and-error approach.

WORKFLOW OF IMAGE-GUIDED SPINE SURGERY AND CASE ILLUSTRATION

A 65-year-old female had a previous open laminectomy for L4-5 spinal stenosis within the past 5 years. She currently had mechanical back pain with right L5 radiculopathy and was diagnosed with L4-5 spondylolisthesis with foraminal stenosis. She was planned for minimally invasive extraforaminal lumbar interbody fusion L4-5 with an expandable cage under intraoperative 3D CT navigation guidance. Preoperative images are shown in **Fig. 9**.

Preoperative Planning

Before proceeding with surgery, a comprehensive review of the patient's recent clinical presentation and radiographic images, along with their correlation is crucial. In cases where intraoperative CT is unavailable, the preoperative CT dataset can be transferred to the navigation system, allowing for preoperative planning of the pedicle screws' direction, size, and length with the navigation software. However, it is important to keep in mind that positional changes may lead to some accuracy issues. To minimize navigation errors from patient movement, it is generally recommended to administer general anesthesia during the procedure.

Positioning and Operation Room Setup

Positioning
The patient is positioned on the radiolucent table, with a cushion placed under the pressure area. To maintain a secure patient position, adhesive tape should be utilized. For cervical procedures, the Mayfield skull clamp system is recommended for stability.

Operation room setup
The layout of the operating room is illustrated in **Fig. 10**. The gantry of the intraoperative CT scanner is positioned on the cranial side of the table, located between the anesthesiologist staff and the operative table. The surgeon typically stands on the affected side of the patient, while the assistant stands on the opposite side. The scrub nurse and instrument table are positioned caudally. The navigation monitor, infrared camera arm, and control unit are placed at the caudal end of the table. In cases where electromagnetic-based navigation is utilized, the electromagnetic field generator is positioned around the patient's gluteal area to generate the electromagnetic field within the surgical working area.

Navigation setup, image acquisition, and registration
Various bony spots are feasible to fix the reference array to the patient securely, including the ilium,

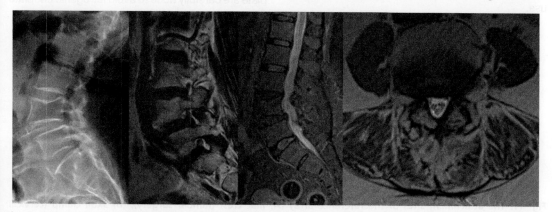

Fig. 9. Preoperative images revealed L4-5 spondylolisthesis with foraminal stenosis and previous laminectomy.

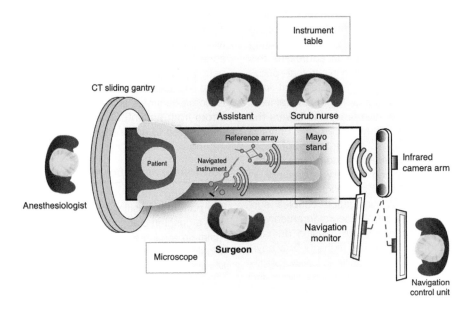

Fig. 10. Layout of the operative room and navigation unit.

spinous process, or skull clamp in cervical spine surgery. However, it is essential that the reference array is placed in close proximity to the surgical working area to allow for continuous signal transmission to the navigation infrared camera throughout the entire procedure (**Fig. 11**A-B). At the start of the operation, intraoperative CT images of the surgical region are obtained, and a 3D reconstruction is generated. To prevent radiation exposure to the surgical staff, all personnel exit the operating room while a radiology technician initiates the scan remotely using a control outside the room. The acquired images are automatically transferred and registered with the navigation system. The surgeon performs verification of the navigation instrument. Once these steps are completed, the navigation system is ready for use.

Operation with Intraoperative 3D CT Navigation Guidance

Navigational guidance can be utilized for every step of the procedure, as a "Total navigation principle". Navigation pointer is used to determine the skin incision for percutaneous screw placement (**Fig. 12**). Placement of percutaneous pedicle screws is performed under navigation guidance to identify the proper screw trajectory, size, and length (**Fig. 13**). A separate fascial incision is made and the muscles are dilated to place a table-mounted tubular retractor for an extraforaminal approach. Partial lateral facetectomy is performed to identify the disc level and decompress the exiting nerve root under microscope with nerve stimulation (**Fig. 14**).

Discectomy and preparation of the vertebral endplate are carefully done to avoid iatrogenic endplate

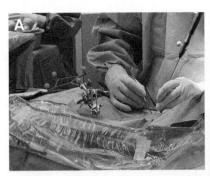
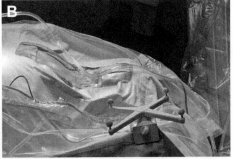

Fig. 11. The attachment sites of the reference array (*A*) Iliac crest (lumbar surgery), (*B*) Skull clamp (cervical surgery).

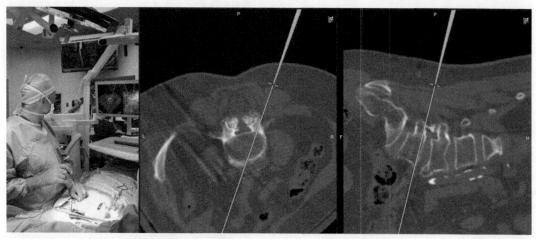

Fig. 12. Skin incision and screw trajectory planning.

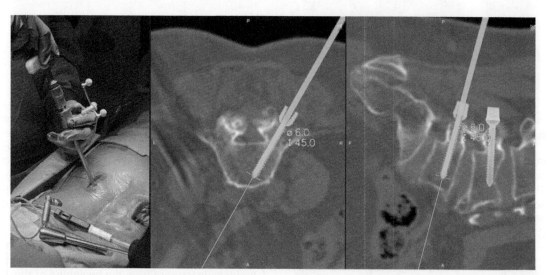

Fig. 13. Percutaneous pedicle screw placement. Direction, size, and length of the screws can be adjusted by findings of intraoperative CT navigation.

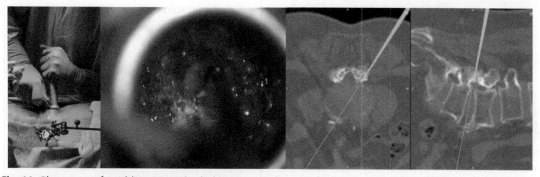

Fig. 14. Placement of a table-mounted tubular retractor for extraforaminal approach and partial lateral facetectomy to identify the disc and decompression of exiting nerve root.

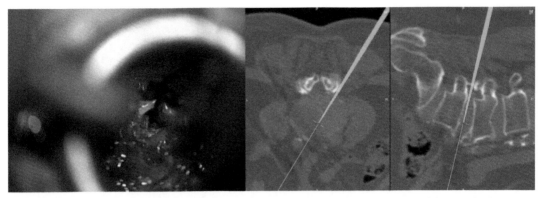

Fig. 15. Discectomy and endplate preparation. The optimal size, direction, and position of the interbody cage can be planned under CT navigation.

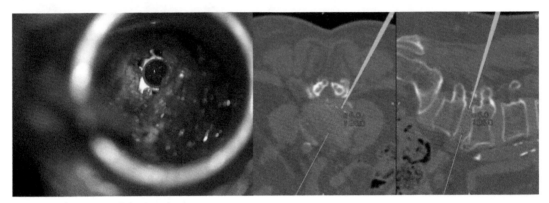

Fig. 16. Implantation of the interbody cage.

injury (**Fig. 15**). An expandable cage packed with bone graft is implanted under navigation guidance. The cage is expanded under surgeon's control to achieve endplate-to-endplate fit to restore disc height and lordosis (**Fig. 16**). A final intraoperative CT scan is obtained to confirm position of pedicular

screws and cage, adequacy of decompression, and optimal cage expansion (**Fig. 17**).

CLINICS CARE POINTS

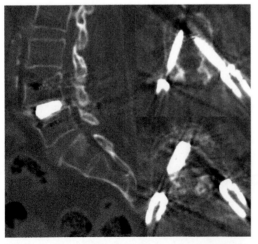

Fig. 17. Intraoperative CT images after decompression, screw placement, and interbody cage implantation revealed optimal instrument position and reduction of spondylolisthesis.

Problem: Inaccuracy from the beginning of the procedure

Pitfalls

- Positional change or movement after image acquisition
- Significant spinal alignment change in prone compared to supine position (preoperative CT image dataset)
- Inadequate stability of reference array fixation (eg, poor bone quality, incomplete bone purchase, spinous process fracture from overtightening of the reference array attachment)

Pearls

- Tape the patient securely in both transverse and longitudinal direction to the operating table to minimize movement
- Verify several anatomic landmarks

- Obtain intraoperative CT if available
- Use curvature correction software
- Obtain stable fixation of the reference array with a secure bone purchase or attach the reference array to the skull clamp for cervical surgery
- Conventional fluoroscopy should be available as a backup in case of uncorrectable navigation failure.

Problem: Inaccuracy during the operation

Pitfalls

- Deflection of the reference array
- Spinal alignment changes during procedure (eg, patient movement, disc height or lordosis increase after cage implantation)
- Attach the reference array too distant from surgical area

Pearls

- Beware of inadvertently hitting the reference array or positional change of the patient
- Repeat image acquisition and verification if inaccuracy is suspect
- Reposition the array fixation point to be closer to surgical area and repeat registration

Problem: Unawareness of inaccuracy

Pitfalls

- Solely rely on navigational image without awareness of possible inaccuracy problem

Pearls

- Comprehensive knowledge of the anatomy is essential.
- Recognize the tactile feedback from surgical instrument and correlate with the navigational images
- Re-verification of navigation accuracy after any forceful action is applied such as after aggressive use of mallet
- Take intraoperative CT scan to verify implant accuracy before closure

Problem: Poor navigation signal

Pitfalls

- The tracking camera is either not facing the reference array or positioned too far away.
- Line-of-sight interruptions
- Contamination of reflective spheres from blood stain or soft tissue debris

Pearls:

1. Correctly reposition the tracking camera

   - Remove the obstacles in the line-of-sight and clean the reflective spheres

RECENT TECHNOLOGIES ON SPINAL NAVIGATION AND FUTURE PERSPECTIVES

Technological advancements have significantly enhanced spinal navigation, making it more beneficial, safe, and user-friendly. The integration of software intelligence has played a crucial role in supporting navigation technology and offering valuable toolsets for improved clinical outcomes.

One of these useful features is CT-MRI image fusion which allows for co-registration of CT images with preoperative MRI scans. CT imaging excels in providing high-resolution views of bony structures, while MRI offers detailed insights into soft tissues such as nerves, intervertebral discs, blood vessels, and soft tissue tumors. The integration of both image types enables surgeons to navigate through these intricate anatomic structures with greater precision and confidence (**Fig. 18A**).[28–30] As previously mentioned, relying solely on imported preoperative images for intraoperative navigation can lead to reduced accuracy due to potential changes in spinal alignment. To address this issue, curvature correction software has been developed, which facilitates the fusion of preoperative and intraoperative images (see **Fig. 18B**). This innovative software corrects the image dataset in the operating room and compensates for the changing spinal alignment to provide an updated anatomic position during navigation.

Software intelligence has also contributed much to the advancement of image-guide spine surgery (see **Fig. 18C**). Such software enables surgeons to meticulously plan every step of the procedure before entering the operating room. This includes defining the optimal placement of pedicle screws, designing rod contours, determining the size and angle for osteotomy to correct deformities, positioning interbody cages, and accurately identifying tumor volume and boundaries. To expedite the planning process, the software incorporates automated labeling or segmentation of vertebral levels (see **Fig. 18D**).

The development of image-guided technology has been a significant driving force behind the growth of navigation-based technology, marking a crucial step toward incorporating other advanced technologies, such as augmented reality (AR) and robotics into the field of spine surgery. Augmented reality can significantly assist spine surgery by integrating navigational images to display surgical anatomy or target pathologies by projecting images onto the surgeon's head-mounted goggles or through a microscope-mediated heads-up display.[31] The high accuracy achieved through intraoperative navigation has paved the way for the development of robotic-assisted spine surgery.

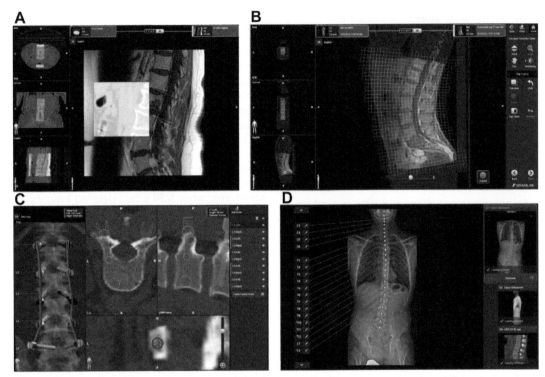

Fig. 18. Software intelligence enhancing spinal navigation (Brainlab) (*A*) Co-registration of CT and preoperative MRI image, (*B*) Curvature correction between preoperative and intraoperative images, (*C*) Preoperative planning for screw and rod placement, and (*D*) Automatic level labeling (segmentation). ([*A-D*] With permission from © 2023 Brainlab AG.)

This technology offers surgeons an efficient means of rigid trajectory guidance, relying on precise anatomic registration of the patient's anatomy.[32,33] These groundbreaking innovations will be further discussed in the subsequent chapters, promising to revolutionize the future of spine surgery and enhance patient outcomes.

SUMMARY

Image-guided navigation in spine surgery is a cutting-edge technology that revolutionizes how we approach complex spinal procedures. This advanced system combines real-time imaging data with precise location tracking device. While no technology can fully replace the clinical expertise and skill of an experienced spine surgeon, navigation systems offer valuable benefits by providing a comprehensive view of surgical anatomy, allowing surgeons to perform surgery with greater precision while reducing radiation exposure. Various navigation systems are currently available and continuously evolving to improve surgical precision and outcomes in spine surgery. Furthermore, image-guided navigation serves as a foundation for incorporating other advanced technologies like AR and robotics into spine surgery.

DISCLOSURE

The Authors have nothing to disclose.

REFERENCES

1. Mao JZ, Agyei JO, Khan A, et al. Technologic Evolution of Navigation and Robotics in Spine Surgery: A Historical Perspective. World Neurosurg 2021;145:159–67.
2. Fehlings MG, Ahuja CS, Mroz T, et al. Future Advances in Spine Surgery: The AOSpine North America Perspective. Neurosurgery 2017;80(3s):S1–s8.
3. Hussain I, Cosar M, Kirnaz S, et al. Evolving Navigation, Robotics, and Augmented Reality in Minimally Invasive Spine Surgery. Global Spine J 2020;10(2 Suppl):22S–33S.
4. Otomo N, Funao H, Yamanouchi K, et al. Computed Tomography-Based Navigation System in Current Spine Surgery: A Narrative Review. Medicina (Kaunas). 2022;58(2).
5. Garcia-Fantini M, De Casas R. Three-dimensional fluoroscopic navigation versus fluoroscopy-guided placement of pedicle screws in L4-L5-S1 fixation:

single-centre experience of pedicular accuracy and S1 cortical fixation of 810 screws. J Spine Surg 2018;4(4):736–43.

6. Costa F, Cardia A, Ortolina A, et al. Spinal navigation: standard preoperative versus intraoperative computed tomography data set acquisition for computer-guidance system: radiological and clinical study in 100 consecutive patients. Spine (Phila Pa 1976) 2011;36(24):2094–8.

7. Sommer F, Goldberg JL, McGrath L Jr, et al. Image Guidance in Spinal Surgery: A Critical Appraisal and Future Directions. Int J Spine Surg 2021;15(s2): S74–86.

8. Yao Y, Jiang X, Wei T, et al. A real-time 3D electromagnetic navigation system for percutaneous pedicle screw fixation in traumatic thoraco-lumbar fractures: implications for efficiency, fluoroscopic time, and accuracy compared with those of conventional fluoroscopic guidance. Eur Spine J 2022; 31(1):46–55.

9. Sagi HC, Manos R, Benz R, et al. Electromagnetic field-based image-guided spine surgery part one: results of a cadaveric study evaluating lumbar pedicle screw placement. Spine 2003;28(17): 2013–8.

10. Fraser JF, Von Jako R, Carrino JA, et al. Electromagnetic navigation in minimally invasive spine surgery: results of a cadaveric study to evaluate percutaneous pedicle screw insertion. SAS J 2008;2(1): 43–7.

11. Hagan MJ, Remacle T, Leary OP, et al. Navigation Techniques in Endoscopic Spine Surgery. BioMed Res Int 2022;2022:8419739.

12. Koivukangas T, Katisko JP, Koivukangas JP. Technical accuracy of optical and the electromagnetic tracking systems. SpringerPlus 2013;2(1):90.

13. von Jako R, Finn MA, Yonemura KS, et al. Minimally invasive percutaneous transpedicular screw fixation: increased accuracy and reduced radiation exposure by means of a novel electromagnetic navigation system. Acta Neurochir 2011;153(3): 589–96.

14. Xu DR, Luan LR, Ma XX, et al. Comparison of electromagnetic and optical navigation assisted Endo-TLIF in the treatment of lumbar spondylolisthesis. BMC Musculoskelet Disord 2022;23(1):522.

15. von Jako RA, Carrino JA, Yonemura KS, et al. Electromagnetic navigation for percutaneous guide-wire insertion: accuracy and efficiency compared to conventional fluoroscopic guidance. Neuroimage 2009; 47(Suppl 2):T127–32.

16. Kalfas IH. Image-guided spinal navigation: application to spinal metastases. Neurosurg Focus 2001; 11(6):e5.

17. Marintschev I, Gras F, Klos K, et al. Navigation of vertebro-pelvic fixations based on CT-fluoro matching. Eur Spine J 2010;19(11):1921–7.

18. Rajasekaran S, Bhushan M, Aiyer S, et al. Accuracy of pedicle screw insertion by AIRO((R)) intraoperative CT in complex spinal deformity assessed by a new classification based on technical complexity of screw insertion. Eur Spine J 2018;27(9):2339–47.

19. Kim TT, Drazin D, Shweikeh F, et al. Clinical and radiographic outcomes of minimally invasive percutaneous pedicle screw placement with intraoperative CT (O-arm) image guidance navigation. Neurosurg Focus 2014;36(3):E1.

20. Shin BJ, James AR, Njoku IU, et al. Pedicle screw navigation: a systematic review and meta-analysis of perforation risk for computer-navigated versus freehand insertion. J Neurosurg Spine 2012;17(2): 113–22.

21. Matityahu A, Kahler D, Krettek C, et al. Three-dimensional navigation is more accurate than two-dimensional navigation or conventional fluoroscopy for percutaneous sacroiliac screw fixation in the dysmorphic sacrum: a randomized multicenter study. J Orthop Trauma 2014;28(12):707–10.

22. Matur AV, Palmisciano P, Duah HO, et al. Robotic and navigated pedicle screws are safer and more accurate than fluoroscopic freehand screws: a systematic review and meta-analysis. Spine J 2023; 23(2):197–208.

23. Hiyama A, Katoh H, Nomura S, et al. Intraoperative computed tomography-guided navigation versus fluoroscopy for single-position surgery after lateral lumbar interbody fusion. J Clin Neurosci 2021;93: 75–81.

24. Tan BH, Sockalingam S, Ganesan D. The use of intraoperative CT navigation for posterior cervical spine foraminotomy. Br J Neurosurg 2023;1–4.

25. McGrath LB Jr, Kirnaz S, Goldberg JL, et al. Microsurgical Tubular Resection of Intradural Extramedullary Spinal Tumors With 3-Dimensional-Navigated Localization. Oper Neurosurg (Hagerstown) 2022; 23(4):e245–55.

26. Mendelsohn D, Strelzow J, Dea N, et al. Patient and surgeon radiation exposure during spinal instrumentation using intraoperative computed tomography-based navigation. Spine J 2016;16(3):343–54.

27. Leitner L, Bratschitsch G, Sadoghi P, et al. Navigation versus experience: providing training in accurate lumbar pedicle screw positioning. Arch Orthop Trauma Surg 2019;139(12):1699–704.

28. Tabarestani TQ, Sykes DAW, Maquoit G, et al. Novel Merging of CT and MRI to Allow for Safe Navigation into Kambin's Triangle for Percutaneous Lumbar Interbody Fusion-Initial Case Series Investigating Safety and Efficacy. Oper Neurosurg (Hagerstown) 2023;24(3):331–40.

29. Rawicki N, Dowdell JE, Sandhu HS. Current state of navigation in spine surgery. Ann Transl Med 2021; 9(1):85.

30. Yamanaka Y, Kamogawa J, Katagi R, et al. 3-D MRI/CT fusion imaging of the lumbar spine. Skeletal Radiol 2010;39(3):285–8.

31. Jitpakdee K, Liu Y, Heo DH, et al. Minimally invasive endoscopy in spine surgery: where are we now? Eur Spine J 2023;32(8):2755–68.

32. Lopez IB, Benzakour A, Mavrogenis A, et al. Robotics in spine surgery: systematic review of literature. Int Orthop 2023;47(2):447–56.

33. Rasouli JJ, Shao J, Neifert S, et al. Artificial Intelligence and Robotics in Spine Surgery. Global Spine J 2021;11(4):556–64.

Functional Stimulation and Imaging to Predict Neuromodulation of Chronic Low Back Pain

Timothy J. Florence, MD, PhD, Ausaf Bari, MD, PhD, Andrew C. Vivas, MD*

KEYWORDS

- Chronic low back pain • Neuromodulation • Deep brain stimulation • Chronic pain
- Pain centralization

KEY POINTS

- Conscious perception of mechanical, claudicatory, and radicular pain relies on distinct neuroanatomical substrates.
- Spine surgery classically targets peripheral generators, but pain can centralize through plasticity in ascending pathways and brain sensory–affective networks.
- Patients with centralized pain may be good candidates for neuromodulation.

INTRODUCTION

Although it is said that *pain is an illusion*, it may be more correct to say that pain is an emergent phenomenon; that is, the subjective perception of pain represents a construction of the central nervous system to assign both meaning and context to aversive sensory signals and coordinate behavioral responses to them. Chronic low back pain (cLBP) is perhaps the single most common source of disability worldwide. Understanding cLBP in the context of the neurobiology of pain stands to improve patient selection for traditional surgery versus neuromodulation.

Dysfunction of nearly every tissue time within the spine—muscle, vertebra, joint, disk, or neuronal—can contribute to back pain. Central to the traditional philosophy of spine surgery is the belief that focusing on treating the peripheral source of pain will result in clinical benefit. Unfortunately, an experience well known to spine surgeons is the patient suffering from severe back pain without radiographic pathology. Furthermore, there is growing acceptance that certain types of pain may be refractory to even the most technically sound spinal procedures. One potential explanation for this phenomenon is the idea that pain perception depends not only on sensation at the periphery but on the significant modulatory influences of cognitive and affective brain processing. In this context, all central brain substrates involved in the processing of back pain become potential sites for maladaptive changes via a process loosely termed "pain centralization." Importantly, these foci also become candidate sites for therapeutic intervention.

Spinal cord stimulation (SCS) may still be too peripheral. Emerging work has identified both anatomic changes and therapeutic targets in brains of patients with refractory severe cLBP. In this present work, we describe a framework for understanding back pain in the context of central pain pathways. We trace how aversive interoceptive signals travel from the musculoskeletal and peripheral neuronal components of the spine to produce the conscious perception of pain. We will describe current understanding of central brain alterations in patients with refractory back pain and discuss contemporary and emerging treatment options in treating patients with centralized back pain.

UCLA Neurosurgery, 300 Stein Plaza Driveway, Suite 562, Los Angeles, CA 90095, USA
* Corresponding author.
E-mail address: avivas@mednet.ucla.edu

Neurosurg Clin N Am 35 (2024) 191–197
https://doi.org/10.1016/j.nec.2023.11.004
1042-3680/24/© 2023 Elsevier Inc. All rights reserved.

BACK PAIN: FROM THE PERIPHERY TO PREFRONTAL CORTEX

Spine surgeons are highly familiar with the multifactorial nature of back pain. They may be less familiar, however, with how such pain is encoded by the nervous system. Pain qualities (eg, mechanical, claudicatory, and radicular pain) are transduced via distinct mechanisms. Mechanical back pain, whether muscular, discogenic, or facetogenic, is thought to be conveyed by branches of the posterior primary sensory ramus.[1] Medial branches of this nerve famously innervate the local segmental facet as well as multifidus muscle. Anatomic studies demonstrate some degree of adjacent segmental innervation as well. Intermediate and lateral branches innervate longissimus and iliocostalis, respectively. Disk space innervation is complex (**Fig. 1**). The anterior and lateral disk space of the cephalad and caudal segment is innervated by branches of the sympathetic chain. The recurrent sinuvertebral nerve forms from the coalescence of gray rami and direct sensory branches to innervate the posterior and posterolateral portions of the proximal and cephalad disk space via projection through the spinal canal. Nociceptive free nerve endings have been observed in periosteum, cancellous bone, facet capsule, and penetrate into disk annulus.[2] Electrophysiologic and immunohistochemical studies suggest that these represent a heterogenous population driven by nociceptive signaling peptides, including calcitonin gene related peptide (CGRP), substance P, and isolectin B (IB)4[3,4] and are further modulated by inflammatory cytokines tumor necrosis factor (TNF)-a, interleukin (IL)-6, and IL-8.[5] Mounting evidence supports a role for detection of mechanical pain by directly mechanosensitive channels, such as Piezo2,[6,7] TrpC,[8] and ASIC3.[9]

Claudicatory back pain, on the other hand, likely represents a mixed disorder of compression, neuronal perfusion, and altered metabolism. Canal diameter compromise from lipomatosis, facet hypertrophy, ligamentum flavum hypertrophy and calcification, or disk degeneration raise both local thecal cerebrospinal fluid[10,11] and venous pressures.[12] This local pressure exists at rest but is exacerbated by activity.[13] The correlation of neurogenic claudication with physical activity may result from local reduction in nerve perfusion pressure exacerbated by reduced nerve metabolite clearance by cerebrospinal fluid pulsation. Ischemic pain is transduced by chemosensitive neurons expressing receptors to detect the byproducts of anaerobic metabolism: local acidosis, adenosine diphosphate (ADP),[14] and heat.[15] This mechanistically links ischemia and nociception.

In contrast, mechanical compression of the dorsal root ganglion is the proximal cause of radicular pain. Preceding the Hodgkin–Huxley model by nearly 2 decades,[16] early pathologic descriptions of disk herniation proposed prolongation of sensory transmission as the underlying mechanism of radicular pain.[17] To date, it is well established that dual insults of inflammation and compression of the dorsal root ganglion or its proximal root produce ectopic activity in A-delta and C-fibers perceived as lancinating pain.[18] This evidence results in part from experiments in which lumbosacral dorsal root ganglion (DRG) was forcibly compressed in awake patients with forceps or temporary suture,[19,20] reproducing sharp pain in a dermatomal distribution. Despite a conceptually simple etiology, dorsal root ganglion compression produces a complex cascade of secondary effects.[21] Ectopic activity mediated by voltage-gated sodium channels seems to underlie the electric "shooting" sensation,[22] whereas inflammation mediated by TNF-a and chemokines IL-1 and IL-6 are likely responsible for ongoing smoldering pain and soreness.[23] Curiously, the least well-characterized effect is the etiology of dermatomal numbness which may be a result of elevated signaling threshold, sensory neuronal apoptosis, or lateral inhibition.[24,25]

How does back pain reach consciousness? Peripheral pain signals travel as electrical impulses along nociceptive A-delta and C-fibers to the dorsal horn of spinal gray matter. Individual neurons canonically synapse in superficial layers of the Rexed lamina, the substantia gelatinosa, and the nucleus proprius.[26]

Second-order neurons decussate locally and ascend cranially. The primary ascending nociceptive pathway is the anterolateral spinothalamic tracts.[27] Supplementary ascending pathways include the spinoreticular and spinomesencephalic tracts. The spinoreticular tract may play an

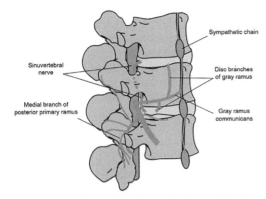

Fig. 1. Innervation of the thoracolumbar axial spine.

Sympathetic chain

Sinuvertebral nerve

Disc branches of gray ramus

Medial branch of posterior primary ramus

Gray ramus communicans

important role in carrying collateral information to the limbic system; the spinomesencephalic tract is thought to drive activity of brain stem endogenous analgesic centers.[28,29] Indeed, first-order synapses are dense with mu- and kappa-opioid receptors. This highlights that foci for modulation, whether endogenous or exogenous, are distributed throughout the pain system.

At third-order synapses, neuroanatomical segregation of thalamic and extrathalamic relays support the processing of distinct pain features. Sensory percepts or the discriminative properties of pain, such as intensity, location, and duration, are processed via synapses in somatosensory cortex. Evaluative features, such as pain significance or its relation to recent behavior, are supported by white matter projections to areas critical for attention, memory, and decision-making such as prefrontal cortex and hippocampus. Emotional aspects of pain, including fear and anxiety, may be assigned by activity in anterior cingulate cortex, insula, and the amygdala among other distributed networks.

Descending influence modulates pain information before it reaches cortex.[26] Prefrontal cortex and limbic nuclei both drive activity in periaqueductal gray (PAG) and rostroventromedial medulla, which have been shown to attenuate pain signals as distal as the dorsal horn. In a remarkable series of fMRI experiments in human patients, spinal BOLD signal was shown to be modulated by the anticipation of pain, directly experiencing it, and placebo anesthesia.[30–32] Both ascending and descending pathways play an important and direct role in the subjective experience of pain.

ALTERATIONS

The underlying assumption in spine surgery is that symptom relief will be achieved by targeting and treating the initial peripheral origin of the pain. However, pathologic change anywhere along canonical pain pathways can lead to subjective sensory experiences of pain independent of inciting stimuli. Pain centralization describes a heterogeneous set of pain syndromes in which pain generation moves centripetally.[33] Initially recognized in the context of physical therapy,[34] it is associated with poor treatment prognosis.[35] Pain centralization is likely multifactorial phenomena due in part to differences in stress response, psychological sensitivities, and changes to the nervous system.

Chronic back pain is specifically associated with widespread structural and functional changes to the brain.[36–39] As may be predicted by its neuroanatomical substrate, affected areas subserve limbic, reward, and somatosensory functions. Replicated volumetric studies in living human patients have revealed gray matter decrements in dorsolateral prefrontal cortex, temporal lobes, insula, somatosensory cortex, and cuneus. Both increases and decreases in gray matter volume have been reported in the anterior cingulate, amygdala, basal ganglia, and thalamus.[40–43] Alterations in white matter are somewhat controversial; however, decline of white matter volume has been reported in the corpus callosum and anterior limb of the internal capsule.[41,44]

Although structural changes demonstrate variable results, functional studies are remarkably consistent. First, chronic back pain is associated with widespread changes in default mode network, or resting-state connectivity, of the brain.[45,46] Increased activity is observed in medial prefrontal cortex, cingulate cortex, amygdala, and insula, even at rest. Provoking maneuvers seem to drive activity in dorsolateral prefrontal cortex, insula, motor cortex, and anterior cingulate. Somatosensory cortex may encode specific spatiotemporal features of pain quality: differential S1 activity has been observed following movement, pain exacerbating movement, and high versus low pain conditions.[47–51]

Intriguingly, evidence suggests that patients with chronic low back pain show differential responses to other aversive stimuli.[52] Mechanical stimuli induce enhanced activity in orbitofrontal cortex, somatosensory cortex, posterior cingulate, and insula, whereas PAG activity was diminished compared with normal controls. Aversive thermal stimuli led to enhanced responses in medial prefrontal cortex and insula; moreover, activity in nucleus accumbens alone can be used to discriminate if a patient suffers from chronic low back pain. In summary, the unique responses of patients with quality of life altering chronic low back pain may reflect broad differences in aversive stimuli encoding.

NEUROMODULATORY STRATEGIES

Patients in whom pain generation has been suspected to have migrated several synapses from the periphery should be considered for neuromodulation. Although this population has been historically challenging for the spine surgeon, the continuous technological evolution today allows for tailored, patient-specific neuromodulatory strategies to address refractory pain. It is conceptually useful to think of these strategies as targeted to specific sites of putative pain centralization.

Neuromodulatory therapy for pain has ancient roots: ancient Egyptians, Greeks, and Romans applied electrogenic catfish, torpedo fish, and eels to the body to produce anesthesia.[53–57] In the intervening millenia, tools have evolved such that there are now several options to target back pain of central origin. SCS is one such option. Originally thought to use sensory gating of noxious stimuli,[58] the therapeutic mechanism of SCS remains poorly understood and may rely on autonomic[59] or supratentorial effects.[60] Perhaps best characterized in the context of treating refractory extremity pain (eg, complex regional pain syndrome), it has also been studied as a treatment for surgically refractory back pain.[61] Although smaller patient series have shown encouraging results, outcomes have been less extraordinary in larger subsequent studies.[62–64] Further, recent meta-analyses have raised questions about the duration of therapeutic benefit.[65] Still, trial implantation remains a reasonable intervention to offer patients who suffer medically refractory pain with equivocal structural abnormality.

Brain targets have also been investigated. Described in small series using off-label application of deep brain stimulation (DBS) systems, these include PAG, periventricular gray, ventral posterolateral nucleus (VPL)/ventral posteromedial (VPM) thalamus, and anterior cingulate cortex. Modulation has also been targeted to internal capsule (anterior or posterior limb), septal nuclei, posterior hypothalamus, and nucleus accumbens. As suggested by their position as relays in parallel pain processing pathways, modulating activity is directed toward modifying distinct features of pain. Efficacy is difficult to determine in absolute terms; however, roughly 70% of patients receiving PAG-DBS for back pain in one experimental trial opted to proceed with system internalization.[66,67] While encouraging, replication with larger cohorts is necessary to rigorously evaluate how well these targets treat chronic low back pain.

Modulating network activity, rather than focal nuclei, represents an emerging strategy in the treatment of centralized back pain. Our group is particularly interested in the subgenual cingulate cortex (SCC) as a target to alter broad networks involved in the divergent encoding of nociceptive internal states. Subgenual cingulate (SCC), or Area 25, was initially investigated as a DBS target for depression. Depression and refractory back pain are not only comorbid conditions. There is increasing evidence that they are subserved by shared network substrate. We believe that there is significant promise in modulating this particular network hub toward alleviating centralized back pain, even in the case of distributed representation.[36] We have recently implanted the first in human bilateral SCC for cLBP, with good preliminary results (Ausaf Bari, personal communication, 2023) **(Fig. 2)**.

FUTURE DIRECTIONS

Optimal outcomes are achieved when intervention is tailored to pain generation. To date, spine surgeons do so by careful synthesis of clinical history, physical examination, and careful radiographic review. Still, these efforts may be foiled by centralized pain. How can one predict with certainty which patients will respond to spinal surgery, and which patients will require neuromodulation, from clinical data alone? We believe in a future in which assigning equivocal patients to spinal surgery or modulatory therapy will be informed by direct neurophysiological measurement. As we have reviewed before, fMRI has revealed fundamentally distinct responses to aversive stimuli in patients suffering from cLBP versus healthy controls. Further, it is sensitive enough to detect endogenous descending neuromodulatory influences in the case of chronic pain. It remains to be seen which of these imaging biomarkers, if any, can differentiate surgical responders from nonresponders. Patient selection based on objective neurobiologic assessment would constitute a holy grail for all physicians treating patients with chronic pain, including spine surgeons.

Two emerging technologies show significant promise in this regard. The first is functional ultrasound, which is capable of detecting activity-associated neurovascular coupling of small blood

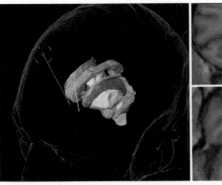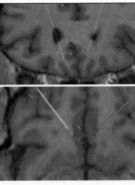

Fig. 2. Localization of DBS leads within the Subgenual Cingulate Cortex for Chronic Low back Pain.

vessels. The applications of functional ultrasound have already been explored in brain-awake tumor surgery, where it has been used as a type of hand-held hyperlocal fMRI.[68,69] Such a system could be used to monitor activity in dorsal columns, superficial Rexed laminae, and anterolateral fibers to tailor surgical decompression or assess intraoperatively therapeutic response to SCS. Second, functional neurosurgeons developing closed-loop neuromodulatory techniques have explored invasive intracranial depth electrode monitoring to identify idiosyncratic modulatory targets on a tailored patient basis.[70] Depression is thought to share neuroanatomical substrate with chronic low back pain, and similar treatment strategies could be conceptually extended to this population. Definitive but invasive localization would be reserved for patients who have failed multiple lines of therapy.

SUMMARY

Understanding the anatomy of chronic back pain, from source to cerebrum, is crucial to implementing effective treatment strategies. Here, we have explored how distinct qualities of back pain are transduced by unique mechanisms at the periphery, how these signals travel along afferent paths to the brain, and how divergent brain pathways represent subsets of painful percepts. Surgical intervention on the axial spine can be an effective treatment for pain generation. However, it may fail in the setting of subjective pain experience being generated by pathologic change at higher order synapses.

It is precisely these patients who should be directed toward neuromodulatory modalities. Thankfully, interventions exist to target pathologic pain encoding at many synapses: from peripheral nerves, to ascending sensory signals, to deep brain nuclei. Promising technologies on the horizon may harbinger a day in which optimal therapeutic intervention is steered by objective neurophysiologic measurement and imaging biomarkers. Until that day, precise diagnosis of pain generators may be improved by a firm understanding of the neurobiological basis of back pain.

CLINICS CARE POINTS

- Back pain, such as all sensory percepts, relies on fundamental processes like sensory transduction, lateral inhibition, and descending modulation.
- Spine surgery treats peripheral pain generation.

- Patients with centralized pain may be best treated with tailored neuromodulatory strategies.
- Emerging technologies may allow for neurophysiologically based therapy selection.

DISCLOSURE

TJ Florence reports no conflicts. A. Bari is a principal investigator for study NIH UH3 NS111136, Deep Brain Stimulation of the Subgenual Cingulate Cortex for the Treatment of Medically Refractory Chronic Low Back Pain. A. C. Vivas is a consultant for Nuvasive and ATEC and receives funding as a Casa Colina Rehabilitation Center Fellow.

REFERENCES

1. Cavanaugh JM, Ozaktay AC, Yamashita HT, et al. Lumbar facet pain: biomechanics, neuroanatomy and neurophysiology. J Biomech 1996;29(9):1117–29.
2. Hurri H, Karppinen J. Discogenic pain. Pain 2004; 112(3):225–8.
3. Ashton IK, Roberts S, Jaffray DC, et al. Neuropeptides in the human intervertebral disc. J Orthop Res 1994;12(2):186–92.
4. Nencini S, Ivanusic JJ. The physiology of bone pain. how much do we really know? Front Physiol 2016;7. https://doi.org/10.3389/fphys.2016.00157.
5. Solovieva S, Leino-Arjas P, Saarela J, et al. Possible association of interleukin 1 gene locus polymorphisms with low back pain. Pain 2004;109(1–2): 8–19.
6. Coste B, Mathur J, Schmidt M, et al. Piezo1 and Piezo2 are essential components of distinct mechanically activated cation channels. Science 2010;330(6000):55–60.
7. Eijkelkamp N, Linley JE, Torres JM, et al. A role for Piezo2 in EPAC1-dependent mechanical allodynia. Nat Commun 2013;4:1682.
8. Chen CC, Wong CW. Neurosensory mechanotransduction through acid-sensing ion channels. J Cell Mol Med 2013;17(3):337–49.
9. Ohtori S, Inoue G, Koshi T, et al. Up-regulation of acid-sensing ion channel 3 in dorsal root ganglion neurons following application of nucleus pulposus on nerve root in rats. Spine 2006;31(18):2048–52.
10. Magnaes B. Clinical recording of pressure on the spinal cord and cauda equina. Part 1: the spinal block infusion test: method and clinical studies. J Neurosurg 1982;57(1):48–56.
11. Magnaes B. Clinical recording of pressure on the spinal cord and cauda equina. Part 2: position changes in pressure on the cauda equina in central lumbar spinal stenosis. J Neurosurg 1982;57(1): 57–63.

12. Porter RW. Spinal stenosis and neurogenic claudication. Spine 1996;21(17):2046–52.

13. Kim HJ, Kim H, Kim YT, et al. Cerebrospinal fluid dynamics correlate with neurogenic claudication in lumbar spinal stenosis. PLoS One 2021;16(5):e0250742.

14. Queme LF, Ross JL, Lu P, et al. Dual Modulation of Nociception and Cardiovascular Reflexes during Peripheral Ischemia through P2Y1 Receptor-Dependent Sensitization of Muscle Afferents. J Neurosci 2016;36(1):19–30.

15. Caterina MJ, Leffler A, Malmberg AB, et al. Impaired nociception and pain sensation in mice lacking the capsaicin receptor. Science 2000;288(5464):306–13.

16. Hodgkin AL, Huxley AF. A quantitative description of membrane current and its application to conduction and excitation in nerve. J Physiol 1952;117(4):500–44.

17. Mixter WJ, Barr JS. Rupture of the Intervertebral Disc with Involvement of the Spinal Canal. N Engl J Med 1934;211(5):210–5.

18. Merskey H. Clarifying definition of neuropathic pain. Pain 2002;96(3):408–9.

19. Norlén JG, Ray EA. On the Value of the Neurological Symptoms in Sciatica for the Localization of a Lumbar Disc Herniation. A Contribution to the Problem of the Surgical Treatment of Sciatica.Translated by Edward Adams-Ray.; 1944.

20. Smyth MJ, Wright V. Sciatica and the intervertebral disc; an experimental study. J Bone Joint Surg Am 1958;40-A(6):1401–18.

21. Lin JH. Lumbar radiculopathy and its neurobiological basis. World J Anesthesiol 2014;3(2):162.

22. Olmarker K, Rydevik B, Hansson T, et al. Compression-induced changes of the nutritional supply to the porcine cauda equina. J Spinal Disord 1990;3(1):25–9.

23. Su YS, Sun WH, Chen CC. Molecular mechanism of inflammatory pain. World J Anesthesiol 2014;3(1):71–81.

24. Beggs S, Salter MW. Stereological and somatotopic analysis of the spinal microglial response to peripheral nerve injury. Brain Behav Immun 2007;21(5):624–33.

25. Colburn RW, Rickman AJ, DeLeo JA. The effect of site and type of nerve injury on spinal glial activation and neuropathic pain behavior. Exp Neurol 1999;157(2):289–304.

26. Willis WD, Westlund KN. Neuroanatomy of the pain system and of the pathways that modulate pain. J Clin Neurophysiol 1997;14(1):2–31.

27. Almeida TF, Roizenblatt S, Tufik S. Afferent pain pathways: a neuroanatomical review. Brain Res 2004;1000(1–2):40–56.

28. Bourne S, Machado AG, Nagel SJ. Basic anatomy and physiology of pain pathways. Neurosurg Clin N Am 2014;25(4):629–38.

29. De Broucker T, Cesaro P, Willer JC, et al. Diffuse noxious inhibitory controls in man. Involvement of the spinoreticular tract. Brain 1990;113(Pt 4):1223–34.

30. Eippert F, Finsterbusch J, Bingel U, et al. Direct evidence for spinal cord involvement in placebo analgesia. Science 2009;326(5951):404.

31. Wager TD, Rilling JK, Smith EE, et al. Placebo-induced changes in FMRI in the anticipation and experience of pain. Science 2004;303(5661):1162–7.

32. Tinnermann A, Geuter S, Sprenger C, et al. Interactions between brain and spinal cord mediate value effects in nocebo hyperalgesia. Science 2017;358(6359):105–8.

33. Donelson R, Silva G, Murphy K. Centralization phenomenon. Spine 1990;15(3):211–3.

34. McKenzie RA, May S. The lumbar spine. Mechanical diagnosis & therapy 1981;1:374.

35. Werneke M, Hart DL. Centralization phenomenon as a prognostic factor for chronic low back pain and disability. Spine 2001;26(7):758–64. ; discussion 765.

36. Kashanian A, Tsolaki E, Pouratian N, et al. Deep brain stimulation of the subgenual cingulate cortex for the treatment of chronic low back pain. Neuromodulation 2022;25(2):202–10.

37. Kregel J, Meeus M, Malfliet A, et al. Structural and functional brain abnormalities in chronic low back pain: A systematic review. Semin Arthritis Rheum 2015;45(2):229–37.

38. Ng SK, Urquhart DM, Fitzgerald PB, et al. The relationship between structural and functional brain changes and altered emotion and cognition in chronic low back pain brain changes: a systematic review of MRI and fMRI studies. Clin J Pain 2018;34(3):237–61.

39. Nijs J, Clark J, Malfliet A, et al. In the spine or in the brain? Recent advances in pain neuroscience applied in the intervention for low back pain. Clin Exp Rheumatol 2017;35(5):108–15.

40. Fritz HC, McAuley JH, Wittfeld K, et al. Chronic back pain is associated with decreased prefrontal and anterior insular gray matter: results from a population-based cohort study. J Pain 2016;17(1):111–8.

41. Buckalew N, Haut MW, Morrow L, et al. Chronic pain is associated with brain volume loss in older adults: preliminary evidence. Pain Med 2008;9(2):240–8.

42. Wasan AD, Loggia ML, Chen LQ, et al. Neural correlates of chronic low back pain measured by arterial spin labeling. Anesthesiology 2011;115(2):364–74.

43. Dolman AJ, Loggia ML, Edwards RR, et al. Phenotype matters: the absence of a positive association between cortical thinning and chronic low back pain when controlling for salient clinical variables. Clin J Pain 2014;30(10):839–45.

44. Čeko M, Shir Y, Ouellet JA, et al. Partial recovery of abnormal insula and dorsolateral prefrontal connectivity to cognitive networks in chronic low back pain after treatment. Hum Brain Mapp 2015;36(6): 2075–92.

45. Pijnenburg M, Brumagne S, Caeyenberghs K, et al. Resting-state functional connectivity of the sensorimotor network in individuals with nonspecific low back pain and the association with the sit-to-stand-to-sit task. Brain Connect 2015;5(5):303–11.

46. Kornelsen J, Sboto-Frankenstein U, McIver T, et al. Default mode network functional connectivity altered in failed back surgery syndrome. J Pain 2013;14(5): 483–91.

47. Kong J, Spaeth RB, Wey HY, et al. S1 is associated with chronic low back pain: a functional and structural MRI study. Mol Pain 2013;9:43.

48. Yu R, Gollub RL, Spaeth R, et al. Disrupted functional connectivity of the periaqueductal gray in chronic low back pain. Neuroimage Clin 2014;6: 100–8.

49. Loggia ML, Kim J, Gollub RL, et al. Default mode network connectivity encodes clinical pain: an arterial spin labeling study. Pain 2013;154(1):24–33.

50. Baliki MN, Baria AT, Apkarian AV. The cortical rhythms of chronic back pain. J Neurosci 2011; 31(39):13981–90.

51. Berger SE, Baria AT, Baliki MN, et al. Risky monetary behavior in chronic back pain is associated with altered modular connectivity of the nucleus accumbens. BMC Res Notes 2014;7:739.

52. Giesecke T, Gracely RH, Grant MAB, et al. Evidence of augmented central pain processing in idiopathic chronic low back pain. Arthritis Rheum 2004;50(2): 613–23.

53. Panagiotis T, Efthimios S, Vasilis G, et al. Neuromodulation and chronic pain. Published 2008. http://e-journal.gr/wp/wp-content/uploads/pdf/2008/4.%20Neuromodulation%20and%20Chronic%20Pain.pdf. Accessed August 31, 2023.

54. Goroszeniuk T, Pang D. Peripheral neuromodulation: a review. Curr Pain Headache Rep 2014;18(5):412.

55. Deer TR, Esposito MF, McRoberts WP, et al. A systematic literature review of peripheral nerve stimulation therapies for the treatment of pain. Pain Med 2020;21(8):1590–603.

56. van Gorp EJJAA, Teernstra OPM, Gültuna I, et al. Subcutaneous stimulation as ADD-ON therapy to spinal cord stimulation is effective in treating low back pain in patients with failed back surgery syndrome: a multicenter randomized controlled trial. Neuromodulation 2016;19(2):171–8.

57. McRoberts WP, Wolkowitz R, Meyer DJ, et al. Peripheral nerve field stimulation for the management of localized chronic intractable back pain: results from a randomized controlled study. Neuromodulation 2013;16(6):565–74. discussion 574-5.

58. Melzack R, Wall PD. Pain mechanisms: a new theory. Science 1965;150(3699):971–9.

59. Kemler MA, Barendse GA, van Kleef M, et al. Spinal cord stimulation in patients with chronic reflex sympathetic dystrophy. N Engl J Med 2000;343(9): 618–24.

60. Meyerson BA, Linderoth B. Mechanisms of spinal cord stimulation in neuropathic pain. Neurol Res 2000;22(3):285–92.

61. Frey ME, Manchikanti L, Benyamin RM, et al. Spinal cord stimulation for patients with failed back surgery syndrome: a systematic review. Pain Physician 2009;12(2):379–97.

62. Eldabe SS, Taylor RS, Goossens S, et al. A Randomized Controlled Trial of Subcutaneous Nerve Stimulation for Back Pain Due to Failed Back Surgery Syndrome: The SubQStim Study. Neuromodulation 2019;22(5):519–28.

63. North RB, Ewend MG, Lawton MT, et al. Failed back surgery syndrome: 5-year follow-up after spinal cord stimulator implantation. Neurosurgery 1991;28(5): 692–9.

64. Kumar K, Taylor RS, Jacques L, et al. Spinal cord stimulation versus conventional medical management for neuropathic pain: a multicentre randomised controlled trial in patients with failed back surgery syndrome. Pain 2007;132(1–2):179–88.

65. Traeger AC, Gilbert SE, Harris IA, et al. Spinal cord stimulation for low back pain. Cochrane Database Syst Rev 2023;3(3):CD014789.

66. Boccard SGJ, Pereira EAC, Aziz TZ. Deep brain stimulation for chronic pain. J Clin Neurosci 2015; 22(10):1537–43.

67. Coffey RJ. Deep brain stimulation for chronic pain: results of two multicenter trials and a structured review. Pain Med 2001;2(3):183–92.

68. Claron J, Hingot V, Rivals I, et al. Large-scale functional ultrasound imaging of the spinal cord reveals in-depth spatiotemporal responses of spinal nociceptive circuits in both normal and inflammatory states. Pain 2021;162(4):1047–59.

69. Urban A, Dussaux C, Martel G, et al. Real-time imaging of brain activity in freely moving rats using functional ultrasound. Nat Methods 2015;12(9): 873–8.

70. Xiao J, Provenza NR, Asfouri J, et al. Decoding Depression severity from intracranial neural activity. Biol Psychiatry 2023. https://doi.org/10.1016/j.biopsych.2023.01.020.

Advances in Anterolateral Approaches to the Lumbar Spine
A Focus on Technological Developments

Rohit Prem Kumar, BA[a], Galal A. Elsayed, MD[b], Daniel M. Hafez, MD, PhD[c], Nitin Agarwal, MD[a],*

KEYWORDS

- Spinal surgery • Anterolateral approaches • Intraoperative image guidance • Robotics
- Augmented reality • Machine learning

KEY POINTS

- Anterolateral approaches to the spine have undergone significant advances in the past few decades.
- Advances in intraoperative imaging, such as three-dimensional (3D) imaging and computer-assisted navigation, have demonstrated advantages for patients and surgeons.
- Technologies such as robotics, augmented reality, and machine learning show great potential but require careful evaluation.

HISTORICAL PERSPECTIVES

The history of spine surgery has been a continual journey of innovation and adaptation, driven by the relentless pursuit to better the human condition. Early documented treatments for spine pathology date back to the sixteenth century BC with accounts of the cervical spine and associated cord injury management by Egyptian priests, the physicians of that era. Simply put, the prescription was rest, bandages, and dressings.[1] It was only two millennia later that the first surgical intervention of the spine was reported.[2] This article discusses the technological advances since then, particularly related to anterolateral approaches to spine surgery. The term anterolateral encompasses anterior, lateral, and oblique approaches.

Anterior Approach

In 1906, Müller documented one of the earliest anterior approaches to the lumbar spine. Müller attempted to use a transperitoneal approach to excise a tuberculosis abscess of the spine (ie, Pott's disease). Unfortunately, the procedure did not have favorable outcomes overall and was abandoned.[3] Nonetheless, Norman Capener built on this approach in 1932 and described the anterior lumbar interbody fusion (ALIF). In 1960, Paul Harmon revised Capener's ALIF procedure to use an extraperitoneal approach instead of a transperitoneal approach. In particular, this procedure was employed for those patients who had already failed two or more posterior surgeries.[4] Harmon demonstrated satisfactory outcomes, even at a 12-year

a Department of Neurological Surgery, University of Pittsburgh School of Medicine, UPMC Presbyterian, Suite B-400, 200 Lothrop Street, Pittsburgh, PA 15213, USA; b Och Spine, Weill Cornell Medicine/NewYork-Presbyterian, 525 East 68th Street, New York, NY 10068, USA; c Department of Neurosurgery, Washington University School of Medicine in St. Louis, 660 South Euclid Avenue, Campus Box 8057, St. Louis, Missouri 63110, USA
* Corresponding author. Department of Neurological Surgery, University of Pittsburgh Medical Center, 200 Lothrop Street, Suite B-400, Pittsburgh, PA 15213.
E-mail address: nitin.agarwal@upmc.edu

Neurosurg Clin N Am 35 (2024) 199–205
https://doi.org/10.1016/j.nec.2023.11.006
1042-3680/24/© 2023 Elsevier Inc. All rights reserved.

follow-up.[4] Despite Harmon's efforts early on, the ALIF remained controversial.[3]

However, in 1997, the ALIF was reinvigorated by Michael Mayer with the introduction of his mini-open approach. The new approach reduced operative time and resulted in less trauma to the patient.[5] The mini-open ALIF also became the seed for the lateral and oblique approaches that followed in the decades after.[3]

The anterior approach to the spine is achieved by making an incision in the lower abdomen, moving aside the abdominal viscera, and carefully retracting the abdominal vasculature in front of the spine. This creates a corridor that allows direct access to the disc space and avoids direct manipulation of the spinal nerves, reducing the risk of nerve injury.[6] In its current form, the ALIF allows surgeons to achieve maximal disc space visualization and consequentially maximize the implant footprint. To this end, endplate subsidence can be minimized.[7] For degenerative disc disease, the stand-alone ALIF has been shown to have better clinical and radiographic outcomes, reduced operative time, and blood loss compared to conventional posterior approaches.[8] In addition, the ALIF demonstrates adequate clinical and radiographic outcomes for spinal deformity. However, there remains a 13% overall complication rate.[7,9,10] Complications include vascular injury, abdominal organ injury, and retrograde ejaculation.[11]

Lateral Approach

Despite the advances of the ALIF, there was still a need for less traumatic approaches to the spine. This need was met by Luiz Pimenta in 2006 with his pioneering of the lateral lumbar interbody fusion (LLIF). The patient is placed in the lateral decubitus position. The surgeon makes an incision in the side of the patient's torso before traversing through the psoas muscle to the intervertebral disc. This retroperitoneal, transpsoas approach avoids the great vessels, thecal sac, and spinal nerve roots.[12] Furthermore, the LLIF does not require a general or vascular surgeon for access as the norm for spine surgeons employing the ALIF approach. Moreover, the incision is smaller, and there is earlier postoperative patient mobilization.[11] In addition, the LLIF with posterior spinal fusion (PSF) is superior to conventional PSF techniques (ie, TLIF and PLIF) in clinical and radiographic improvements without differences in complication rates.[13,14]

However, the LLIF has its limitations. These limitations include difficulty accessing the L5-S1 disc space, increased lumbar plexus injury risk, psoas muscle trauma, and reliance on neuromonitoring.[11,15] Furthermore, using the procedure in isolation may not be ideal in cases with severe central canal stenosis, bony lateral recess stenosis, and high-grade spondylolisthesis.[11]

Oblique Approach

The anterior-to-psoas technique (ATP), also known as the oblique lateral interbody fusion (OLIF), was introduced to address the limitations of the LLIF.[3] The ATP is a retroperitoneal, ante-psoas method to access the lumbar spine. In this approach, the patient is situated in the lateral decubitus position, and a slightly ventral incision is created to grant entry into the retroperitoneal space. The psoas muscle is gently retracted aside and safeguarded instead of being penetrated. The disc space can then be visualized.[16,17] The benefits of this approach included shorter operative times and reduced risk of injuring the psoas muscle and nearby nerves, with some reports citing a lower incidence of transient and permanent weakness (1% vs 3%) compared to the LLIF.[18]

Additionally, the ATP can be performed at the L5-S1 disc level, which, in essence, is an ALIF performed in the lateral position. This approach allows access to the traditional ALIF corridor but with the benefits of a lateral/anterolateral approach. Evidence in the current literature shows that stand-alone ATP is safe and effective for mild to moderate adult spinal deformity.[19] Additionally, it may allow greater sagittal deformity correction without needing a posterior subtraction osteotomy, although further studies are needed to confirm this.[15,20,21]

Nevertheless, the ATP has several associated risks, such as a higher rate of vascular complications than the LLIF (2% vs <0.5%). Other risks include abdominal ileus from manipulation of the retroperitoneal space and numbness or weakness in the psoas or quadriceps muscles from excessive muscle retraction.[16] Overall, there is still a high incidence of intraoperative (4.9%) and postoperative (29.6%) complications.[19]

TECHNOLOGICAL INNOVATIONS
Interbody Cages

There have been significant developments in cage technology that have translated to improved postoperative outcomes. One example is the introduction of the polyetheretherketone (PEEK) cage in the 1990s, which allowed surgeons to address the issue of cage subsidence. Subsidence refers to the phenomenon whereby the operated disc space decreases postoperatively.[22] This occurs when the cage sinks into the vertebral body leading to several clinical implications such as loss of spinal alignment, persistent or recurrent symptoms of pain, instability, and in severe cases, neurologic symptoms due to compression.[23] PEEK cages have been reported to have similar fusion rates as solid titanium cages but with decreased subsidence rates.[23]

On the contrary, studies have also indicated that titanium cages have superior fusion and subsidence rates.[24,25] In particular, three-dimensional (3D) printed porous titanium (pTi) cages were approved in 2017 and have been shown to yield lower subsidence rates than PEEK.[26] This is partly due to the low modulus of elasticity of pTi, which is closer to the modulus of elasticity of native bone than solid titanium.[27]

Apart from making pTi viable, 3D printing has revolutionized interbody graft technology by making patient-specific cages a reality. Spine surgeons can order cages that are customized specifically for the anatomy of each patient and that can distribute the load more evenly due to increased contact area.[28] There is weak evidence that this translates to potentially superior subsidence and pseudarthrosis rates. However, patient-specific cages are estimated to cost two to five times more than off-the-shelf cages. Additionally, it may take up to two to four weeks for the production of a patient-specific cage.[29]

Another significant advancement in interbody cage technology has been the hyperlordotic cage for complex spinal deformity surgery. Correction of severe spinal deformities has traditionally been from the posterior approach using the posterior subtraction osteotomy (PSO).[30] However, the PSO is a particularly morbid procedure with a complication rate of up to 58% (11% of which is neurologic), mean estimated blood loss of 1.1 L, and high rates of pseudarthrosis. Hyperlordotic cages allow similar lordosis correction but with drastically reduced complication rates (21% overall and 4.1% neurologic) and blood loss (240 mL) in combination with the ALIF.[30] Moreover, hyperlordotic cages can overpower prior posterior spinal instrumentation to restore lumbar lordosis in patients with pseudarthrosis.[31]

Intraoperative Image Guidance

Intraoperative image guidance has significantly improved the accuracy of surgical procedures such as pedicle screw fixation. Posterior fixation is often used with LLIF and ATP procedures, especially in cases demonstrating abnormal preoperative dynamic motion.[32] Some suggest that intraoperative image guidance for screw placement yields fewer complications and improved clinical measures.[33] One advancement in the intraoperative imaging realm was the introduction of 3D fluoroscopic imaging which showed significantly higher screw placement accuracy (95.5%) than conventional fluoroscopy (68.1%) or two-dimensional (2D) fluoroscopy (84.3%).[34] An additional downside of conventional fluoroscopy is the continuous radiation exposure to the patient and surgical staff. This has been effectively addressed with computer-assisted navigation in which an apparatus utilizes stereotactic cameras to track instruments in 3D space. This is then overlayed with a computed tomography (CT) or MRI image to generate a map that can guide instrumentation.[33] In a single-center study comparing navigation with conventional fluoroscopy for the ATP, there was no difference in operative time, estimated blood loss, length of hospitalization, or perioperative complications. However, there was significantly less radiation in the navigation group (which a single CT image) than in the fluoroscopy group (which used several X-rays). However, the authors noted that the opposite may be true at centers where fewer fluoroscopy images are captured.[35]

Robotics

The accuracy of surgical procedures can be further enhanced using robotic assistance. Robotic assistance has been shown to place pedicle screws with improved accuracy and yield decreased average length of stay for patients.[36] Regarding anterolateral approaches, studies have investigated the utility of robots for percutaneous PSF in the lateral position while performing single-position LLIF and ATP. Single-position LLIF and ATP eliminate the need for patient repositioning, reducing the risk of injury and operative time.[37,38] However, percutaneous PSF is difficult in the lateral position. Some initial studies showed that robotic assistance increased the safety and accuracy of percutaneous PSF in this position.[39,40] However, a systematic review by Patel and colleagues found no significant difference in pedicle screw placement accuracy with robotic assistance compared to conventional techniques.[39] Aside from pedicle screw fixation, there is limited literature on using robots for anterior, lateral, and oblique approaches to the spine. Case series have been published reporting fusion rates, complication rates, and clinical and radiographical outcomes for robot-assisted ALIFs that are comparable to the mini-open ALIF.[41,42] Despite the feasibility and safety of robot-assisted ALIF, large-scale studies need to be conducted before widespread adoption. Furthermore, small-scale studies need to be undertaken to evaluate robot-assisted approaches to the LLIF and ATP.

Spatial Computing

Despite the promise of robotics for surgery, there exist multiple limitations, including a lack of tactile feedback, misplacement of pedicle screws due to skiving, and the exorbitant cost of purchasing a robot (often over $1,000,000).[43] In addition, other advancements, such as computer-assisted navigation, also pose challenges, including interruption of the surgeon's workflow due to line of sight disturbances and attention displacement.[44]

Spatial computing (SC) devices seek to bypass the challenges of robotics and computer-assisted navigation. One subtype of SC is augmented reality (AR) which, in the spine, generally works by overlaying 3D reconstructions of the spine on the surgeon's view, generating a "see-through effect."[45] Although there is limited literature on the effectiveness of AR devices for spine surgery, a recent dual-center prospective study examined the use of AR devices for pedicle screw placement supplementing ALIFs and LLIFs. The study found that the accuracy of screw placement with AR was comparable to screw placement with a robot. Additionally, the intraoperative screw revision rate was 0.49%, and no instrumentation was revised postoperatively.[46]

Virtual reality (VR) is another subtype of SC. In VR, the surgeon's entire environment is computer-generated.[45] VR allows the surgeon to assess musculature, ligaments, abdominal viscera, and neurovasculature preoperatively and plan the trajectory appropriately. Postoperatively, VR allows surgeons to assess the placement of instrumentation and changes in radiographic parameters.[47] However, a drawback of VR is that it cannot be used intraoperatively.[47] Additionally, an obstacle common to AR and VR use is the physical discomfort (eg, vertigo and headaches) associated with head-mounted devices.[45] Moreover, as with AR, there is limited literature on the effectiveness of VR.

Machine Learning

Machine learning is increasingly being used to optimize outcomes, particularly in the field of surgery. Prior to surgical procedures, machine learning can assist in conducting a comprehensive risk-benefit analysis. By analyzing large volumes of data from similar previous cases, these algorithms can provide accurate predictions regarding patient-specific outcomes, such as the potential complications and expected improvement in quality of life measures. Such data-driven insights can significantly enhance point-of-care decision-making and facilitate tailored surgical planning.[48] For instance,

Agarwal and colleagues used machine learning to predict surgical outcomes based on body mass index for patients with preoperative obesity and lumbar spondylolisthesis.[49] Additionally, Shahrestani and colleagues utilized machine learning to predict the postoperative length of stay in patients who underwent decompression for spondylolisthesis based on comorbidities, intraoperative factors, and socioeconomic attributes.[50] Moreover, machine learning has begun to find its place in surgical navigation systems through the integration of AR by generating patient-specific 3D reconstructions of the spine based on CT or MRI scans.[51] Overall, the incorporation of machine learning into surgical practice holds great promise for improving patient outcomes and the overall efficiency of health care delivery.

LIMITATIONS

The technologies such as robotics, extended reality, and machine learning covered in this article are still in the early stages of clinical use. The current body of literature on these technologies is relatively limited; as such, additional robust, large-scale studies on these topics are required. Therefore, it is difficult to draw definitive conclusions about their effectiveness and utility based solely on the available literature. Even more so, given the rapid pace of advancements in spinal surgery, the information contained in this article may soon become outdated.

SUMMARY

The field of spine surgery has seen remarkable progress over the centuries, with unprecedented advancements in the last few decades. The evolution of anterolateral approaches to the spine has greatly expanded the surgical armamentarium available for treating spinal pathologies. Modern technological innovations, such as interbody cages, intraoperative image guidance, robotics, augmented reality, and machine learning, have significantly improved surgical outcomes and patient safety. Despite these achievements, challenges and limitations persist, presenting opportunities for further research and development. The future of spine surgery lies in harnessing the full potential of these advancements, addressing the existing limitations, and continuing the trend of patient-centered, outcome-focused innovation. As the understanding of the spine and its pathologies grows and technology advances, the emergence of even more effective and minimally invasive techniques is anticipated.

CLINICS CARE POINTS

- Hyperlordotic cages coupled with the anterior or lateral approaches can yield comparable results to posterior subtraction osteotomy for spinal deformity without the associated morbidity.

- When feasible, computer-assisted navigation should be considered for pedicle screw placement to improve accuracy.

- Robotics, augmented reality, and machine learning for spine surgery are nascent technologies that still require large-scale studies before broader adoption.

STATEMENTS AND DECLARATIONS

Dr N. Agarwal receives royalties from Thieme Medical Publishers and Springer Publishing Company. Dr G.A. Elsayed is the CEO and Co-Founder of Neurite LLC.

REFERENCES

1. Knoeller SM, Seifried C. Historical Perspective: History of Spinal Surgery. Spine 2000;25(21):2838.
2. Smith AG. ARTICLE IX.–Account of a Case in which Portions of Three Dorsal Vertebrae were removed for the relief of Paralysis from Fracture, with partial success. The North American Medical and Surgical Journal (1826-1831) 1829;8(15):94.
3. Matur AV, Mejia-Munne JC, Plummer ZJ, et al. The History of Anterior and Lateral Approaches to the Lumbar Spine. World Neurosurgery 2020;144: 213–21.
4. Harmon Paul H. Anterior extraperitoneal lumbar disk excision and vertebral body fusion. Clin Orthop Relat Res 1960;(18):169–98.
5. Mayer MH. A New Microsurgical Technique for Minimally Invasive Anterior Lumbar Interbody Fusion1996 Scientific Program Committee. Spine 1997;22(6):691.
6. Brau SA. Mini-open approach to the spine for anterior lumbar interbody fusion: description of the procedure, results and complications. Spine J 2002; 2(3):216–23.
7. Rao PJ, Phan K, Giang G, et al. Subsidence following anterior lumbar interbody fusion (ALIF): a prospective study. Journal of Spine Surgery 2017; 3(2):168–75.
8. Udby PM, Bech-Azeddine R. Clinical outcome of stand-alone ALIF compared to posterior instrumentation for degenerative disc disease: A pilot study and a literature review. Clin Neurol Neurosurg 2015;133:64–9.
9. Agarwal N, White MD, Zhang X, et al. Impact of endplate-implant area mismatch on rates and grades of subsidence following stand-alone lateral lumbar interbody fusion: an analysis of 623 levels. J Neurosurg Spine 2020;33(1):12–6.
10. Marchi L, Abdala N, Oliveira L, et al. Radiographic and clinical evaluation of cage subsidence after stand-alone lateral interbody fusion: Clinical article. J Neurosurg Spine 2013;19(1):110–8.
11. Mobbs RJ, Phan K, Malham G, et al. Lumbar interbody fusion: techniques, indications and comparison of interbody fusion options including PLIF, TLIF, MI-TLIF, OLIF/ATP, LLIF and ALIF. J Spine Surg 2015;1(1):2–18.
12. Pawar A, Hughes A, Girardi F, et al. Lateral Lumbar Interbody Fusion. Asian Spine J 2015;9(6):978–83.
13. Yang H, Liu J, Hai Y, et al. What Are the Benefits of Lateral Lumbar Interbody Fusion on the Treatment of Adult Spinal Deformity: A Systematic Review and Meta-Analysis Deformity. Global Spine J 2023; 13(1):172–87.
14. Nayar G, Roy S, Lutfi W, et al. Incidence of adjacent-segment surgery following stand-alone lateral lumbar interbody fusion. J Neurosurg Spine 2021; 35(3):270–4.
15. Woods KRM, Billys JB, Hynes RA. Technical description of oblique lateral interbody fusion at L1–L5 (OLIF25) and at L5–S1 (OLIF51) and evaluation of complication and fusion rates. Spine J 2017; 17(4):545–53.
16. Phan K, Maharaj M, Assem Y, et al. Review of early clinical results and complications associated with oblique lumbar interbody fusion (OLIF). J Clin Neurosci 2016;31:23–9.
17. Silvestre C, Mac-Thiong JM, Hilmi R, et al. Complications and Morbidities of Mini-open Anterior Retroperitoneal Lumbar Interbody Fusion: Oblique Lumbar Interbody Fusion in 179 Patients. Asian Spine J 2012;6(2):89–97.
18. Walker CT, Farber SH, Cole TS, et al. Complications for minimally invasive lateral interbody arthrodesis: a systematic review and meta-analysis comparing pre-psoas and transpsoas approaches. J Neurosurg Spine 2019;30(4):446–60.
19. Zhu L, Wang JW, Zhang L, et al. Outcomes of Oblique Lateral Interbody Fusion for Adult Spinal Deformity: A Systematic Review and Meta-Analysis. Global Spine J 2022;12(1):142–54.
20. Molloy S, Butler JS, Benton A, et al. A new extensile anterolateral retroperitoneal approach for lumbar interbody fusion from L1 to S1: a prospective series with clinical outcomes. Spine J 2016;16(6):786–91.
21. Zairi F, Sunna TP, Westwick HJ, et al. Mini-open oblique lumbar interbody fusion (OLIF) approach for multi-level discectomy and fusion involving L5–S1:

Preliminary experience. J Orthop Traumatol: Surgery & Research 2017;103(2):295–9.

22. Godolias P, Tataryn ZL, Plümer J, et al. Cage subsidence—A multifactorial matter. Orthopädie 2023. https://doi.org/10.1007/s00132-023-04363-9.

23. Seaman S, Kerezoudis P, Bydon M, et al. Titanium vs. polyetheretherketone (PEEK) interbody fusion: Meta-analysis and review of the literature. J Clin Neurosci 2017;44:23–9.

24. Tan JH, Cheong CK, Hey HWD. Titanium (Ti) cages may be superior to polyetheretherketone (PEEK) cages in lumbar interbody fusion: a systematic review and meta-analysis of clinical and radiological outcomes of spinal interbody fusions using Ti versus PEEK cages. Eur Spine J 2021;30(5):1285–95.

25. Alan N, Deng H, Muthiah N, et al. Graft subsidence and reoperation after lateral lumbar interbody fusion: a propensity score-matched and cost analysis of polyetheretherketone versus 3D-printed porous titanium interbodies. J Neurosurg Spine 2023;1–9.

26. Alan N, Vodovotz L, Muthiah N, et al. Subsidence after lateral lumbar interbody fusion using a 3D-printed porous titanium interbody cage: single-institution case series. J Neurosurg Spine 2022; 37(5):663–9.

27. El-Hajje A, Kolos EC, Wang JK, et al. Physical and mechanical characterisation of 3D-printed porous titanium for biomedical applications. J Mater Sci Mater Med 2014;25(11):2471–80.

28. Fernandes RJR, Gee A, Kanawati AJ, et al. Biomechanical Comparison of Subsidence Between Patient-Specific and Non-Patient-Specific Lumbar Interbody Fusion Cages. Global Spine Journal 2022. https://doi.org/10.1177/21925682221134913. 21925682221134910.

29. Wallace N, Schaffer NE, Aleem IS, et al. 3D-printed Patient-specific Spine Implants: A Systematic Review. Clinical Spine Surgery: A Spine Publication. 2020;33(10):400–7.

30. Saville PA, Kadam AB, Smith HE, et al. Anterior hyperlordotic cages: early experience and radiographic results. J Neurosurg Spine 2016;25(6): 713–9.

31. Kadam A, Wigner N, Saville P, et al. Overpowering posterior lumbar instrumentation and fusion with hyperlordotic anterior lumbar interbody cages followed by posterior revision: a preliminary feasibility study. J Neurosurg Spine 2017;27(6):650–60.

32. Blizzard DJ, Thomas JA. MIS Single-position Lateral and Oblique Lateral Lumbar Interbody Fusion and Bilateral Pedicle Screw Fixation. Spine 2018;43(6): 440–6.

33. Rawicki N, Dowdell JE, Sandhu HS. Current state of navigation in spine surgery. Ann Transl Med 2021; 9(1):85.

34. Mason A, Paulsen R, Babuska JM, et al. The accuracy of pedicle screw placement using intraoperative image guidance systems: A systematic review. J Neurosurg Spine 2014;20(2):196–203.

35. Zhang YH, White I, Potts E, et al. Comparison Perioperative Factors During Minimally Invasive Pre-Psoas Lateral Interbody Fusion of the Lumbar Spine Using Either Navigation or Conventional Fluoroscopy. Global Spine J 2017;7(7):657–63.

36. Momin AA, Steinmetz MP. Evolution of Minimally Invasive Lumbar Spine Surgery. World Neurosurgery 2020;140:622–6.

37. Blizzard DJ, Thomas JA. MIS Single-position Lateral and Oblique Lateral Lumbar Interbody Fusion and Bilateral Pedicle Screw Fixation: Feasibility and Perioperative Results. Spine 2018;43(6):440.

38. Ziino C, Konopka JA, Ajiboye RM, et al. Single position versus lateral-then-prone positioning for lateral interbody fusion and pedicle screw fixation. J Spine Surg 2018;4(4):717–24.

39. Patel NA, Kuo CC, Pennington Z, et al. Robot-assisted percutaneous pedicle screw placement accuracy compared with alternative guidance in lateral single-position surgery: a systematic review and meta-analysis. J Neurosurg Spine 2023;1(aop):1–9.

40. Diaz-Aguilar LD, Shah V, Himstead A, et al. Simultaneous Robotic Single-Position Surgery (SR-SPS) with Oblique Lumbar Interbody Fusion: A Case Series. World Neurosurgery 2021;151:e1036–43.

41. Lee Z, Lee JYK, Welch WC, et al. Technique and surgical outcomes of robot-assisted anterior lumbar interbody fusion. J Robotic Surg 2013;7(2):177–85.

42. Beutler WJ, Peppelman WCJ, DiMarco LA. The da Vinci Robotic Surgical Assisted Anterior Lumbar Interbody Fusion: Technical Development and Case Report. Spine 2013;38(4):356.

43. D'Souza M, Gendreau J, Feng A, et al. Robotic-Assisted Spine Surgery: History, Efficacy, Cost, And Future Trends. RSRR 2019;6:9–23.

44. Nottmeier EW. A review of image-guided spinal surgery. J Neurosurg Sci 2012;56(1):35–47.

45. Yoo JS, Patel DS, Hrynewycz NM, et al. The utility of virtual reality and augmented reality in spine surgery. Ann Transl Med 2019;7(Suppl 5):S171.

46. Butler AJ, Colman MW, Lynch J, et al. Augmented reality in minimally invasive spine surgery: early efficiency and complications of percutaneous pedicle screw instrumentation. Spine J 2023;23(1):27–33.

47. Elsayed GA, Lavadi RS, Pugazenthi S, et al. Spatial Computing for preoperative planning and postoperative evaluation of single-position lateral approaches in spinal revision surgery. J Craniovertebral Junction Spine 2023;14(2):208–11.

48. Scheer JK, Smith JS, Schwab F, et al. Development of a preoperative predictive model for major complications following adult spinal deformity surgery. J Neurosurg Spine 2017;26(6):736–43.

49. Agarwal N, Aabedi AA, Chan AK, et al. Leveraging machine learning to ascertain the implications of

preoperative body mass index on surgical outcomes for 282 patients with preoperative obesity and lumbar spondylolisthesis in the Quality Outcomes Database. J Neurosurg Spine 2022;38(2):182–91.

50. Shahrestani S, Chan AK, Bisson EF, et al. Developing nonlinear k-nearest neighbors classification algorithms to identify patients at high risk of increased length of hospital stay following spine surgery. Neurosurg Focus 2023;54(6):E7.

51. Overley SC, Cho SK, Mehta AI, et al. Navigation and Robotics in Spinal Surgery: Where Are We Now? Neurosurgery 2017;80(3S):S86.

Augmented Reality and Virtual Reality in Spine Surgery: A Comprehensive Review

Brendan F. Judy, MD[a],*, Arjun Menta, BS[a], Ho Lim Pak, BS[a],
Tej D. Azad, MD, MS[a], Timothy F. Witham, MD[a]

KEYWORDS

- Augmented reality • Virtual reality • Spine surgery • Navigation • Residency training

KEY POINTS

- Augmented reality and virtual reality are powerful technologies with proven utility and tremendous potential in spine surgery.
- Spine surgery may benefit from these exciting technologies for resident training, preoperative education for patients, surgical planning and execution, and patient rehabilitation.

INTRODUCTION

In the ever-evolving landscape of medical technology, virtual reality (VR) and augmented reality (AR) stand at the forefront of innovative solutions poised to transform health-care delivery. VR, defined as a synthetic environment experienced through computer-generated sensory stimuli, fully immerses the user in a digitally constructed world.[1] This environment, defined by sights, sounds, and tactile feedback (achieved through haptics), is influenced by user interactions, which allow a sense of immersion and manipulation of the environment.[2]

However, AR enhances the user's existing physical environment by superimposing digital information onto the physical world.[3] AR serves as a variant of VR, where the user can manipulate their reality enriched with synthesized sensory information, offering a blend of digital and natural elements.[2] Although some may consider AR and VR as opposites—with AR aiming to augment the real world and VR striving to immerse users in a simulated realm[4]—both hold immense potential to revolutionize various industries, especially medicine.

With the integration of cutting-edge hardware and software, including computerized systems, databases, optical equipment, and robotics, AR/VR have the capability to disrupt industry-standard practices. They open a multitude of opportunities for problem-solving and innovation in the medical field, offering solutions ranging from intricate surgical planning to effective medical training. Spine surgery has developed immense interest in the advent of AR/VR technologies.[5] Both offer a promising avenue to enhance surgical precision, patient safety, and educational efficacy.[6]

This review highlights the importance and impact of AR/VR in spine surgery. It provides insight into the evolution of these technologies, their current platforms and applications in spine surgery, practical uses ranging from preoperative planning to intraoperative navigation, and their role in medical education. Furthermore, it delves into the current challenges, limitations, and future of AR/VR in the field. By offering a comprehensive review of AR/VR, we hope to underscore their potential in enhancing the practice of spine surgery.

EVOLUTION OF AUGMENTED REALITY/VIRTUAL REALITY IN SPINE SURGERY

Early applications of AR and VR systems primarily revolved around diagnosis, training, intraoperative

[a] Department of Neurosurgery, Johns Hopkins Hospital, Johns Hopkins University School of Medicine, 1800 Orleans Street, 6007 Zayed Tower, Baltimore, MD 21287, USA
* Corresponding authors.
E-mail addresses: bjudy1@jhmi.edu (B.F.J.); twitham2@jhmi.edu (T.F.W.)

Neurosurg Clin N Am 35 (2024) 207–216
https://doi.org/10.1016/j.nec.2023.11.010
1042-3680/24/© 2023 Elsevier Inc. All rights reserved.

navigation, and rehabilitation solutions.[7] AR systems have since morphed into 3 principal types: AR surgical navigation, microscope-mediated heads-up display (HUD), and head-mounted display.[8] AR-based microscope HUDs and head-mounted displays have demonstrated benefits in reducing surgeon attention shifting and minimizing line-of-sight visual obstructions when compared with traditional navigation systems.[9]

These groundbreaking solutions have shown utility across several preliminary studies. A meta-analysis conducted in 2022, analyzing 241 patients across 1566 unique reports and 15 publications, revealed enhanced clinical outcomes accompanied by reduced complications and radiation exposure.[10] Another analysis in 2023, incorporating 48 studies assessing VR-assisted training and AR-assisted pedicle screw placement, evidenced benefits in terms of decreased radiation exposure, improved screw placement accuracy, reduced operating time, and lower estimated blood loss compared with traditional techniques.[11] Furthermore, both AR and VR can seamlessly be integrated with other emerging advanced technologies from robotics to wearable technologies.[12]

In addition to the physical technology for visualization, there is immense interest in the innovations revolving around the infrastructure for the integration of AR and VR. A striking example of this is the pipeline developed by Buch and colleagues, which facilitates the generation of 3-dimensional (3D) holographic models during spine surgery for a variety of AR and VR platforms.[13]

Despite these substantial strides, there remains a need for standardization of AR and VR implementation, as well as a more robust clinical data substantiating its utilization and efficacy. As we continue to navigate the era of digital health, the implications and applications of AR and VR in spine surgery are anticipated to grow.

AUGMENTED REALITY/VIRTUAL REALITY TECHNOLOGIES AND PLATFORMS

This section aims to provide an overview of the advantages and limitations of AR and VR. AR tends to be applied more directly to surgical operations, whereas VR finds its niche primarily in patient education and professional training environments.[14] Nevertheless, each brings unique opportunities and equally unique constraints.

Pros

Preoperative Planning and Simulation: Incorporating AR/VR allow physicians to collate information from various sources into a single platform. This facilitates a streamlined preoperative planning process and provides opportunities for practice, approach exploration, and training scenarios that mimic real surgical experiences.

Intraoperative Navigation: AR/VR have been shown to offer substantial benefits in surgical precision and operating room efficiency across a variety of spine surgery procedures, from pedicle screw placement to foraminotomy.[14] Two large case series of AR-assisted pedicle screw placement in consecutive patients reported 98% and 97.7% accuracy.[15,16] AR also has the potential to reduce line-of-sight obstructions, for example, through the utilization of skin markers over the reference frame placement.[17] The integration of AR/VR in robotic-assisted surgery is currently under exploration, with the potential to further mitigate line-of-sight issues and simplify the management of multiple remote screens.

Decreased Radiation Exposure: AR/VR navigation systems can substantially reduce radiation exposure for the surgical team in comparison to fluoroscopy. A 2020 study demonstrated a 32% reduction in effective radiation dose per spinal level treated.[18]

Enhanced Education and Training: AR/VR platforms offer learning tools for surgeons, enabling technical feedback to enhance surgical skills. Studies have shown marked performance improvements and accelerated learning among trainees using AR/VR platforms.[19] These technologies allow for the replication of unique tactile processes, such as dissecting soft tissue or inserting a pedicle screw, thus providing a more realistic training environment compared with nonimmersive simulation[20] and offer preceptors a more objective means of evaluating their trainees' skills.[21]

Cons

Cost: The financial implications of integrating AR/VR, including the costs of the system, power, support infrastructure, development of a hybrid operating room (OR), and equipment maintenance, can be substantial. Currently, there is a lack of comprehensive cost–benefit analyses of AR/VR technologies in the context of spine surgery.

Learning Curve: Proficiency in AR/VR likely requires a time commitment similar to robotic surgery. Looking at robotic surgery as a reference, it is evident that there is a learning curve with one study showing 25 cases to become competent and another demonstrating a consistent decrease in operative time with each additional case.[22,23] Surgeons will have to navigate this to gain the experience and confidence needed to apply these technologies effectively in the operating room. This learning curve represents a potential barrier to adoption and may slow down the rate of integration within spine surgery. However, this is likely to be overcome given the example of robotic surgery adoption.

Battery Life and Comfort: The comfort of the user and the battery life of AR/VR devices are crucial considerations in their design and development. Ergonomic design can significantly affect user experience, and battery life can limit the device's functionality during surgery. Both factors could potentially restrict the adoption of these technologies.

Limited Clinical Data: Several recent large case series have been published, and they demonstrate an excellent safety profile and accurate pedicle screw placement.[15,16,24] Although AR/VR hold immense potential, there is further clinical data needed for evaluating these technologies in spine surgery.[25,26]

The current state of AR/VR used in spine surgery is rapidly evolving. As of June 06, 2023, a range of AR/VR technologies are being used in the field of spine surgery (**Table 1**). The list of these technologies, although not exhaustive, offers an overview of this rapidly evolving landscape, highlighting both the operative and training applications. Awareness of the various technologies and companies behind them are needed in order to promote further evaluation and investigation of their utility.

In summary, the advantages and limitations of AR/VR technologies present a dynamic landscape for further exploration and refinement. As these technologies continue to mature, it is expected that their integration into spine surgery will become more commonplace, with the possibility to improve patient outcomes and potentially revolutionize the surgical field. However, extensive research and development are still necessary to justify and ultimately facilitate widespread adoption.

PREOPERATIVE PLANNING AND SIMULATION

Current preoperative planning and simulation requires analyzing imaging modalities in 2-dimensions (2D). Although these platforms have modernized the approach to neurosurgery and enhanced our understanding of surgical anatomy, they are poorly optimized for translation into the 3D surgical workflow. Typical neuronavigation approximates deeper anatomy by representing it in two 2D planes or one pseudo-3D image with the aid of stereotactic devices on a surgical monitor.[8] Limitations of using this technique include challenges with visualizing deeper anatomy from the perspective of the surgical approach, requiring the surgeon to translate neuronavigational data from a monitor to the actual surgical field; 2D

imaging also lacks real-time visualization of approach during the procedure, requiring additional stereotactic instruments for localization and increasing radiation exposure during the procedure with additional fluoroscopy.

AR/VR attempts to tackle these preoperative challenges to improve surgical planning and simulations. Currently available technologies have approached this in different manners with AR allowing the use of imaging directly overlayed onto the surgical field and VR creating a fully immersive virtual environment outside of the surgical field in which to plan the procedure.[27]

Preoperative or intraoperative imaging is required to create a 3D object that can be used by the AR/VR system. This 3D object is segmented from preoperative imaging scans. Most studies use computed tomography (CT) images to recreate bony anatomy, whereas MRI and PET can also be incorporated into the 3D objects when manipulating soft tissue (eg, tumor biopsy or resection).[27] Because these 3D objects are determined preoperatively by the surgeon, only relevant anatomic structures are isolated. Furthermore, Edstrom and colleagues demonstrated that this process does not add significant duration to the procedure.[18]

Once a 3D object has been created from the preoperative scans, useful information such as route of entry or outlining areas of interests can also be incorporated. This has been particularly useful for pedicle screw placement where the angle of approach can be clearly marked and delineating the maximum extent of resection for spinal tumors.[28] Directly overlaying AR objects therefore obviates the need to approximate the surgical approach and can help less-experienced surgeons visualize deeper anatomy.

AR also allows for accurate fixed anatomic points of reference and may reduce interruption of the surgical workflow. Because the 3D object in AR is typically overlayed onto the patient, calibration of the 3D object with the patient on the surgical table is required. Points of reference that can be identified by both the imaging modality and the camera system are used in most of the institutions. These points for calibration include adhesive skin markers,[17] fiducial markers deeper in the patient such as on bony surface,[13] and reference array attached to the spinous process or posterior superior iliac spine.[29] Manual calibration with voice-commands and hand gestures can also be used with Hololens.[30]

VR allows the surgeon to plan and simulate the procedure away from the operating room. Zheng and colleagues found that using VR to plan the procedure significantly reduced the fluoroscopic time and surgery time while also improving puncture accuracy in endoscopic lumbar discectomy.[31]

Table 1
Current augmented reality/virtual reality technologies in spine surgery

Company	Type	Focus	Application
BrainLab	AR	Operative	• Pedicle screw, cage, and implant placement • Robotic platform integration • Preoperative planning • Reduces radiation exposure
Surgical Theater	AR and VR	Operative/Training	• Surgical navigation • Hardware placement • Preoperative planning • Patient education
Osso VR	VR	Training	• Preoperative planning • Surgical training
Microsoft HoloLens	AR	Operative	• Pedicle screw, cage, and implant placement • Robotic platform integration • Preoperative planning
Augmedics	AR	Operative	• Pedicle screw, cage, and implant placement • Preoperative planning • Reduces radiation exposure
DeGen XR	AR	Training	• Patient education • Surgical training • Preoperative planning
FundamentalVR	VR	Training	• Surgical training
VisAR	AR	Operative	• Pedicle screw, cage, and implant placement • Robotic platform integration • Preoperative planning
Proprio Vision	AR	Operative	• Pedicle screw, cage, and implant placement • Preoperative planning
NextAR	AR	Operative	• Pedicle screw, cage, and implant placement • Preoperative planning • Reduces radiation exposure
LevelEX	AR and VR	Training	• Surgical training • Preoperative planning
7D Surgical	AR	Operative	• Pedicle screw, cage, and implant placement • Preoperative planning • Reduces radiation exposure
Surgalign	AR	Operative	• Pedicle screw, cage, and implant placement • Preoperative planning • Reduces radiation exposure

This table demonstrates an overview of the available AR/VR technologies and applications in spine surgery. Company websites provided a majority of the data.

Moreover, Gasco and colleagues demonstrated that running a VR simulation can significantly improve pedicle screw placement compared with traditional teaching.[32] The use of VR for preoperative planning and simulations can improve surgical decision-making and further reduce surgical complications.

INTRAOPERATIVE NAVIGATION AND VISUALIZATION

Various studies have looked into the benefits of intraoperative navigation and visualization with AR/VR. The main areas that have been assessed include operating time, blood loss, radiation exposure, and accuracy.

In 6 cohort studies that directly compared AR with standard practice, various outcomes among the AR cohort were similar or better than cases using fluoroscopy only.[17,33–37] Although some studies reported a significantly shorter operating time in cases that used AR,[33–35] there is still heterogeneity in operating time reported in the literature.[17,37,36] The shorter operating time may be attributed to the reduced use of intraoperative fluoroscopy due to accurate first-time screw placements. Cases using AR also reported reduced intraoperative blood loss compared to their fluoroscopy-counterparts. Regarding radiation exposure, Gu and colleagues,[33] Auloge and colleagues,[37] Hu and colleagues,[34] and Wei and colleagues[35] reported that AR cases used fluoroscopy fewer times than purely fluoroscopy cases did, which suggests that patients and OR staff were exposed to less radiation. Literature has not reported any significant complication rates or concerns with patient safety among AR cases. In the largest case series to date of 205 consecutively placed pedicle screws (thoracic, lumbar, and sacral) using AR, the accuracy was 98% using the Gertzbein-Robbins scale.[15]

Other benefits of visualization with AR include being able to concurrently visualize the operating field and relevant images using a head-mounted display (**Fig. 1**),[24] a HUD in a surgical microscope,[38] or using a c-arm and monitor.[39] This reduces the amount of attention shifting during the surgery, which can be detrimental for motor and cognitive functions. Additionally, various components of the 3D holographic images can be viewed and removed from view throughout the procedure to further help surgeons to focus on relevant information.

A specific innovative use of AR intraoperatively is in rod bending. Wanivenhaus and colleagues[40] used the camera on the Hololens to create a virtual template for spinal rod implants in phantom models. The authors found that their AR system was quicker than using a pointer-based method at identifying all the screw head centers, significantly reducing the time spent bending and inserting the rod, and significantly improving the accuracy of the rod length.

PREOPERATIVE PATIENT EDUCATION AND POSTOPERATIVE PATIENT REHABILITATION

The use of VR for preoperative patient education has been reported across multiple specialties

with successful reduction in patient anxiety and increased patient understanding of the planned treatment. Radiation oncologists have used a VR smartphone platform to explain radiation therapy to patients with patients reporting increased familiarity and understanding of the therapy procedure.[41] Similarly, cardiac surgeons have reported a significant reduction in patient anxiety when using VR to explain surgery (coronary artery bypass, aortic valve replacement, and thoracic aortic aneurysm repair).[42] Within neurosurgery, Collins and colleagues used VR to explain deep brain stimulation to 30 adult patients and demonstrated increased patient comfort, understanding, and satisfaction.[43] The application of VR to patient education in spine surgery has the potential to improve the patient experience in the clinic and overall increase patient understanding and comfort.

In a similar fashion, VR/AR technology for postoperative assessment and rehabilitation has been explored across various specialties with a particular growing interest since the COVID-19 pandemic.[7,44,45] Such technologies can be used for virtual medical examinations, providing alternative forms of analgesia and enhancing the rehabilitation experience.

With the advent of medical wearable technology and evolving video cameras, virtual monitoring of patients is becoming an easier and viable option.[46] VR systems can be used to virtually assess range of motion of the spine and complete bedside examinations.[48,47] Although various studies have provided guidance for examining patients virtually,[49] there is still a need to create a validated virtual neurologic motor examination.[50]

Studies have shown that the use of VR in pain management can reduce dependence on medication and prevent symptoms of depression.[51] Won and colleagues outlined key characteristics of VR that can act as a distraction therapy and modulate the pain experience.[52] Although there is a scarcity

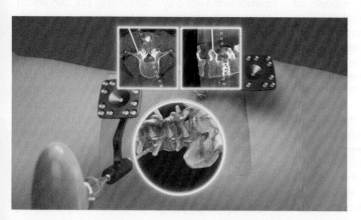

Fig. 1. Intraoperative navigation. Representative image of the surgeon's view through head mounted display in AR-assisted spine surgery. (*Image courtesy* of Augmedics, Inc.)

of literature exploring the use of VR in postoperative spinal cases, current use of VR in nonspine–related orthopedic rehabilitation has demonstrated promising results.[53]

AR/VR have been used in the rehabilitation of patients with various conditions including spinal pathologic conditions and stroke. A review on the use of VR in stroke rehabilitation found that although VR was not better than conventional therapy, it could be useful in improving upper limb function and activities of daily living function when used in addition to standard therapy.[45] Gamification of rehabilitation with VR has been found to be particularly useful for patients recovering from spinal cord injury.[54] Other benefits include being able to provide effective training, being cost-effective and applicable to a broad range of rehabilitation therapy.[51]

Because its use in this area is still in its nascent stage, it is challenging to evaluate the full benefits of AR/VR in rehabilitation because personalized programs have yet to be developed to help patients recover.[55] One barrier of using AR/VR is the upfront cost and accessibility of these devices, whereas cheaper and more ubiquitous gaming consoles may be used instead.[45] Further studies are required to evaluate the benefits of AR/VR in rehabilitation, particularly as to its utility as an adjunct to standard treatments.

SURGEON TRAINING AND EDUCATION

AR/VR offer attractive benefits for neurosurgical training and specifically spine surgery. Spine surgery is performed using many techniques (open, microscopic, endoscopic, percutaneous, and so forth); however, the majority of techniques are performed in a small working space where only 2 surgeons have a view of the operative field. This may limit intraoperative education for trainees. VR allows for a trainee to review the relevant anatomy and the operative plan in a safe space before surgery. Gonzalez-Romo and colleagues[56] conducted a VR simulation of 10 anatomic models of specimens and neurosurgical approaches using Oculus (Meta Platforms, Inc., Menlo Park, CA) and found that 95% of trainees believed this should be a part of neurosurgery training. Chen and colleagues[57] created a VR simulator for lumbar decompression and tested it on 28 trainees. They found that junior trainees had a significant improvement in their anatomic knowledge and understanding of the decompression surgery with the VR simulator. Similar findings were demonstrated in a VR simulator for external ventricular drains with considerable improvement in medical students' accuracy in placement.[58] However, it should be noted that traditional simulators still have their role in education. For example, in one direct comparison of a VR simulator to a physical simulator for endoscopic third ventriculostomy, the physical simulator was superior in teaching dexterity and surgical skills.[59]

In comparison, AR allows for enhanced preoperative and importantly intraoperative learning. Trainees are able to see the intraoperative anatomy with radiological overlay on the surgical field (eg, MRI, CT, and computed tomography angiography [CTA]) in order to comprehend the complex surgical landmarks and corridors. A recent meta-analysis revealed 4 studies on AR systems for spine surgery–specific training.[60] Furthermore, successful in-human AR-assisted instrumentation placement at academic training centers has already been demonstrated in S2-alar-iliac (S2AI) screw placement, spinal oncology, and thoracolumbar fusion, which allows for enhanced resident training.[15,24,61]

Overall, VR allows for preoperative learning and training, whereas AR allows for both preoperative and intraoperative enhanced education. VR simulation may allow for increased access to spine surgery training and level the field of play. In training programs with low volume, AR/VR may supplement the education of trainees. Additionally, these technologies have the capability to provide objective feedback in order to correct technique and transform trainees into surgeons.[21] Finally, AR/VR have the potential to improve training; ultimately, these technologies may lead to improved patient outcomes through superior resident education.

DISCUSSION (CHALLENGES, LIMITATIONS, AND FUTURE DIRECTIONS)

AR/VR have demonstrated successful integration into spine surgery within multiple arenas, including patient education, preoperative and intraoperative education, intraoperative navigation, and postoperative rehabilitation. Ultimately, AR/VR need to demonstrate not only noninferiority but also advantages relative to traditional techniques.

In a cost-conscious market with dwindling spine surgery reimbursements,[62] upfront financial data are needed to validate AR/VR. Although existing data show significant potential of AR/VR in spine surgery, the true question is whether these technologies improve on the current techniques. Several studies[17,33–36] have shown improvement in accuracy of instrumentation or vertebroplasty compared with fluoroscopy, and other studies[15,24] have demonstrated parity of AR-assisted navigation with traditional techniques (freehand, fluoroscopy, CT-navigation, and so forth) in more complex surgery (eg, S2AI and thoracolumbar).

Overall, AR-assisted intraoperative navigation seems safe and accurate. The next step for validation of AR-assisted intraoperative navigation is a more thorough cost analysis comparing AR with existing techniques (robotic, freehand, and fluoroscopy). The AR systems are often significantly cheaper than existing robotic systems and also vendor neutral,[15] which is advantageous. Similar cost-analysis needs to be performed for patient education, resident training, and postoperative rehabilitation in order to determine whether AR/VR are cost-effective. Finally, just as a curriculum has been proposed for robotic spine surgery, a curriculum for AR/VR intraoperative navigation for trainees should be prioritized.[63] This would standardize the training and develop objective measures of competency.

Additionally, studies assessing the patient perspective and outcomes should be performed. Do patients appreciate preoperative education and rehabilitation using AR/VR? Are patient outcomes improved with rehabilitation using AR/VR? How is overall cost affected by AR/VR in spine surgery? These questions deserve thoughtful consideration and payees will demand both financial and clinical outcome data.

SUMMARY

This review highlights the history, current state, and future challenges of AR/VR. AR has successfully integrated into surgical practice through intraoperative navigation. Furthermore, AR/VR have the potential to enhance resident education through simulation and improve intraoperative education with radiological integration. It remains to be seen whether patients and surgeons value these technologies in the preoperative setting as an educational adjunct and postoperatively in the form of rehabilitation. Further work is needed to perform a cost-analysis of AR/VR technology in comparison with existing techniques for patient education and rehabilitation, intraoperative navigation, and resident education.

CLINICS CARE POINTS

- Preoperative
  - Pearls:
    - Streamline preoperative surgical workflow by isolating relevant anatomy on imaging scans, reduce time taken to plan surgical approach, and visualize deeper anatomy
    - Invaluable teaching and learning tool to simulate surgical procedures improve surgical competency
    - Enhanced patient understanding of surgery through simulation
  - Pitfalls:
    - High cost of integrating AR/VR technology, equipment, and hybrid operating room
    - Accurate merging of imaging and identification of anatomic data are needed to create 3D object to overlay on patient anatomy
- Intraoperative
  - Pearls:
    - Improve accuracy of instrumentation placement
    - Reduce operating duration
    - Reduce intraoperative blood loss
    - Reduce intraoperative radiation exposure
    - Enhanced trainee education
  - Pitfalls:
    - Learning curve of using AR/VR technology
    - Cost
- Postoperative
  - Pearls:
    - Improve postoperative pain management and rehabilitation
    - Improve postoperative bedside assessment and examination of patients
  - Pitfalls:
    - Nascent technology that requires constant exploration and improvement
    - Scarcity of literature on postoperative rehabilitation for spine surgery patients

DISCLOSURE

Dr T. F. Witham has received research support from the Gordon and Marilyn Macklin Foundation, United States and is a consultant for, investor in, and is a medical advisory board member for Augmedics. The remaining authors have no disclosures.

REFERENCES

1. Virtual reality. Merriam-Webster Web site. Available at: https://www.merriam-webster.com/dictionary/virtual%

20reality#: ~ :text=noun,what%20happens%20in%20the%20environment. Accessed June 15, 2023.

2. Augmented reality. In: Furht B, editor. Encyclopedia of multimedia. Boston (MA): Springer US; 2006. p. 29–31. https://doi.org/10.1007/0-387-30038-4_10.

3. Augmented reality. Merriam-Webster Web site. Available at: https://www.merriam-webster.com/dictionary/augmented%20reality. Accessed June 15, 2023.

4. Wellner P, Mackay W, Gold R. Computer-augmented environments: Back to the real world. Commun ACM 1993;36(7):24–6.

5. Avrumova F, Lebl DR. Augmented reality for minimally invasive spinal surgery. Front Surg 2023;9:1086988. Available at: https://www.ncbi.nlm.nih.gov/pubmed/36776471.

6. Peters T, Linte C, Yaniv Z, et al. Mixed and augmented reality in medicine. Boca Raton (FL): CRC Press; 2018. p. 304.

7. Yuk FJ, Maragkos GA, Sato K, et al. Current innovation in virtual and augmented reality in spine surgery. Ann Transl Med 2021;9(1):94. Available at: https://www.ncbi.nlm.nih.gov/pubmed/33553387.

8. Barnett GH, Steiner CP, Weisenberger J. Adaptation of personal projection television to a head-mounted display for intra-operative viewing of neuroimaging. J Image Guid Surg 1995;1(2):109–12.

9. Hersh A, Mahapatra S, Weber-Levine C, et al. Augmented reality in spine surgery: A narrative review. HSS J 2021;17(3):351–8. Available at: https://journals.sagepub.com/doi/full/10.1177/15563316211028595.

10. Sumdani H, Aguilar-Salinas P, Avila MJ, et al. Utility of augmented reality and virtual reality in spine surgery: A systematic review of the literature. World Neurosurg 2022;161:e8–17.

11. McCloskey K, Turlip R, Ahmad HS, et al. Virtual and augmented reality in spine surgery: A systematic review. World Neurosurg 2023;173:96–107.

12. Ghaednia H, Fourman MS, Lans A, et al. Augmented and virtual reality in spine surgery, current applications and future potentials. Spine J 2021;21(10):1617–25.

13. Buch VP, Mensah-Brown KG, Germi JW, et al. Development of an intraoperative pipeline for holographic mixed reality visualization during spinal fusion surgery. Surg Innovat 2021;28(4):427–37. Available at: https://journals.sagepub.com/doi/full/10.1177/1553350620984339.

14. Yoo JS, Patel DS, Hrynewycz NM, et al. The utility of virtual reality and augmented reality in spine surgery. Ann Transl Med 2019;7(S5):S171. Available at: https://search.proquest.com/docview/2307153299.

15. Liu A, Jin Y, Cottrill E, et al. Clinical accuracy and initial experience with augmented reality-assisted pedicle screw placement: The first 205 screws. J Neurosurg Spine 2021;1–7. https://doi.org/10.3171/2021.2.SPINE202097.

16. Harel R, Anekstein Y, Raichel M, et al. The XVS system during open spinal fixation procedures in patients requiring pedicle screw placement in the lumbosacral spine. World Neurosurg 2022;164:e1226–32.

17. Elmi-Terander A, Burström G, Nachabe R, et al. Pedicle screw placement using augmented reality surgical navigation with intraoperative 3D imaging: A first in-human prospective cohort study. Spine 2019;44(7):517–25. Available at: https://www.ncbi.nlm.nih.gov/pubmed/30234816.

18. Edstrom E, Burstrom G, Omar A, et al. Augmented reality surgical navigation in spine surgery to minimize staff radiation exposure. Spine 2020;45(1):E45–53.

19. Luciano CJ, Banerjee PP, Bellotte B, et al. Learning retention of thoracic pedicle screw placement using a high-resolution augmented reality simulator with haptic feedback. Neurosurgery 2011;69(3):14–9. Available at: https://www.ncbi.nlm.nih.gov/pubmed/21471846.

20. Shi J, Hou Y, Lin Y, et al. Role of visuohaptic surgical training simulator in resident education of orthopedic surgery. World Neurosurg 2018;111:e98–104.

21. Ponce B, Jennings J, Clay T, et al. Telementoring: use of augmented reality in orthopaedic education: AAOS exhibit selection. J Bone Jt Surg Am Vol 2014;96(10):e84. Available at: http://ovidsp.ovid.com/ovidweb.cgi?T=JS&NEWS=n&CSC=Y&PAGE=fulltext&D=ovft&AN=00004623-201405210-00021.

22. Schatlo B, Martinez R, Alaid A, et al. Unskilled unawareness and the learning curve in robotic spine surgery. Acta Neurochir 2015;157(10):1819–23. Available at: https://link.springer.com/article/10.1007/s00701-015-2535-0.

23. Jiang B, Pennington Z, Azad T, et al. Robot-assisted versus freehand instrumentation in short-segment lumbar fusion: Experience with real-time image-guided spinal robot. World Neurosurg 2020;136:e635–45.

24. Judy BF, Liu A, Jin Y, et al. In-human report of S2 alar-iliac screw placement using augmented reality assistance. Oper Neurosurg (Hagerstown) 2023;24(1):68–73. Available at: https://www.ncbi.nlm.nih.gov/pubmed/36519880.

25. Leger E, Drouin S, Collins DL, et al. Quantifying attention shifts in augmented reality image-guided neurosurgery. Healthc Technol Lett 2017;4(5):188–92.

26. Wachs J. Gaze, posture and gesture recognition to minimize focus shifts for intelligent operating rooms in a collaborative support system. Int J Comput Commun Control 2010;5:106–24.

27. Cho J, Rahimpour S, Cutler A, et al. Enhancing reality: A systematic review of augmented reality in neuronavigation and education. World Neurosurg 2020;139:186–95.

28. Carl B, Bopp M, Sass B, et al. Augmented reality in intradural spinal tumor surgery. Acta Neurochir 2019;161(10):2181–93.

29. Molina CA, Phillips FM, Colman MW, et al. A cadaveric precision and accuracy analysis of augmented reality–mediated percutaneous pedicle implant insertion. J Neurosurg Spine 2021;34(2):316–24. Available at: https://www.ncbi.nlm.nih.gov/pubmed/33126206.

30. Dennler C, Jaberg L, Spirig J, et al. Augmented reality-based navigation increases precision of pedicle screw insertion. J Orthop Surg Res 2020;15(1):174. Available at: https://www.ncbi.nlm.nih.gov/pubmed/32410636.

31. Zheng C, Li J, Zeng G, et al. Development of a virtual reality preoperative planning system for postlateral endoscopic lumbar discectomy surgery and its clinical application. World Neurosurg 2019;123:e1–8.

32. Gasco J, Patel A, Ortega-Barnett J, et al. Virtual reality spine surgery simulation: An empirical study of its usefulness. Neurol Res 2014;36(11):968–73. Available at: https://www.tandfonline.com/doi/abs/10.1179/1743132814Y.0000000388.

33. Gu Y, Yao Q, Xu Y, et al. A clinical application study of mixed reality technology assisted lumbar pedicle screws implantation. Med Sci Mon Int Med J Exp Clin Res 2020;26:e924982. Available at: https://www.ncbi.nlm.nih.gov/pubmed/32647106.

34. Hu M, Chiang C, Wang M, et al. Clinical feasibility of the augmented reality computer-assisted spine surgery system for percutaneous vertebroplasty. Eur Spine J 2020;29(7):1590–6. Available at: https://link.springer.com/article/10.1007/s00586-020-06417-4.

35. Wei P, Yao Q, Xu Y, et al. Percutaneous kyphoplasty assisted with/without mixed reality technology in treatment of OVCF with IVC: A prospective study. J Orthop Surg Res 2019;14(1):255. Available at: https://www.ncbi.nlm.nih.gov/pubmed/31395071.

36. Edström E, Burström G, Persson O, et al. Does augmented reality navigation increase pedicle screw density compared to free-hand technique in deformity surgery? single surgeon case series of 44 patients. Spine 2020;45(17):E1085–90. Available at: https://www.ncbi.nlm.nih.gov/pubmed/32355149.

37. Auloge P, Cazzato RL, Ramamurthy N, et al. Augmented reality and artificial intelligence-based navigation during percutaneous vertebroplasty: A pilot randomised clinical trial. Eur Spine J 2020;29(7):1580–9. Available at: https://link.springer.com/article/10.1007/s00586-019-06054-6.

38. Carl B, Bopp M, Saß B, et al. Microscope-based augmented reality in degenerative spine surgery: Initial experience. World Neurosurg 2019;128:e541–51.

39. Edstrom E, Burstrom G, Nachabe R, et al. A novel augmented-reality-based surgical navigation system for spine surgery in a hybrid operating room: Design, workflow, and clinical applications. Oper Neurosurg (Hagerstown) 2020;18(5):496–502.

40. Wanivenhaus F, Neuhaus C, Liebmann F, et al. Augmented reality-assisted rod bending in spinal surgery. Spine J 2019;19(10):1687–9.

41. Schulz JB, Dubrowski P, Blomain E, et al. An affordable platform for virtual reality-based patient education in radiation therapy. Pract Radiat Oncol 2023. https://doi.org/10.1016/j.prro.2023.06.008.

42. Grab M, Hundertmark F, Thierfelder N, et al. New perspectives in patient education for cardiac surgery using 3D-printing and virtual reality. Front Cardiovasc Med 2023;10:1092007.

43. Collins MK, Ding VY, Ball RL, et al. Novel application of virtual reality in patient engagement for deep brain stimulation: A pilot study. Brain Stimul 2018;11(4):935–7.

44. Berton A, Longo UG, Candela V, et al. Virtual reality, augmented reality, gamification, and tele-rehabilitation: Psychological impact on orthopedic patients' rehabilitation. J Clin Med 2020;9(8):2567. Available at: https://search.proquest.com/docview/2641055706.

45. Laver KE, Lange B, George S, et al. Virtual reality for stroke rehabilitation. Cochrane Database Syst Rev 2017;2018(1):CD008349. Available at: https://www.cochranelibrary.com/cdsr/doi/10.1002/14651858.CD008349.pub4.

46. Morimoto T, Kobayashi T, Hirata H, et al. XR (extended reality: Virtual reality, augmented reality, mixed reality) technology in spine medicine: Status quo and quo vadis. J Clin Med 2022;11(2):470. Available at: https://www.ncbi.nlm.nih.gov/pubmed/35054164.

47. Chang K, Wu W, Chen M, et al. Smartphone application with virtual reality goggles for the reliable and valid measurement of active craniocervical range of motion. Diagnostics 2019;9(3):71. Available at: https://www.ncbi.nlm.nih.gov/pubmed/31295869.

48. Yan C, Wu T, Huang K, et al. The application of virtual reality in cervical spinal surgery: A review. World Neurosurg 2021;145:108–13.

49. Swiatek PR, Weiner JA, Johnson DJ, et al. COVID-19 and the rise of virtual medicine in spine surgery: A worldwide study. Eur Spine J 2021;30(8):2133–42. Available at: https://link.springer.com/article/10.1007/s00586-020-06714-y.

50. Shafi K, Lovecchio F, Forston K, et al. The efficacy of telehealth for the treatment of spinal disorders: Patient-reported experiences during the COVID-19 pandemic. HSS J 2020;16(1_suppl):17–23. Available at: https://journals.sagepub.com/doi/full/10.1007/s11420-020-09808-x.

51. Mishra R, Narayanan MDK, Umana GE, et al. Virtual reality in neurosurgery: Beyond neurosurgical planning. Int J Environ Res Publ Health 2022;19(3):1719. Available at: https://www.ncbi.nlm.nih.gov/pubmed/35162742.

52. Won AS, Bailey J, Bailenson J, et al. Immersive virtual reality for pediatric pain. Children 2017;4(7):52.

Available at: https://www.ncbi.nlm.nih.gov/pubmed/28644422.

53. Gumaa M, Rehan Youssef A. Is virtual reality effective in orthopedic rehabilitation? A systematic review and meta-analysis. Phys Ther 2019;99(10):1304–25. Available at: https://www.ncbi.nlm.nih.gov/pubmed/31343702.

54. Sengupta M, Gupta A, Khanna M, et al. Role of virtual reality in balance training in patients with spinal cord injury: A prospective comparative pre-post study. Asian Spine J 2020;14(1):51–8.

55. Khokale R, S Mathew G, Ahmed S, et al. Virtual and augmented reality in post-stroke rehabilitation: A narrative review. Cureus 2023;15(4):e37559.

56. Gonzalez-Romo NI, Mignucci-Jiménez G, Hanalioglu S, et al. Virtual neurosurgery anatomy laboratory: A collaborative and remote education experience in the metaverse. Surg Neurol Int 2023; 14:90. Available at: https://search.proquest.com/docview/2798711903.

57. Chen T, Zhang Y, Ding C, et al. Virtual reality as a learning tool in spinal anatomy and surgical techniques. N Am Spine Soc J 2021;6:100063.

58. Rossitto CP, Odland IC, Oemke H, et al. External ventricular drain training in medical students improves procedural accuracy and attitudes toward virtual reality. World Neurosurg 2023;175:e1246–54.

59. Breimer GE, Haji FA, Bodani V, et al. Simulation-based education for endoscopic third ventriculostomy: A comparison between virtual and physical training models. Oper Neurosurg (Hagerstown) 2017;13(1): 89–95. Available at: https://www.narcis.nl/publication/RecordID/oai:pure.rug.nl:publications%2F5204d74c-ae60-4643-9c48-f95f0e85db17.

60. Jung Y, Muddaluru V, Gandhi P, et al. The development and applications of augmented and virtual reality technology in spine surgery training: A systematic review. Can J Neurol Sci 2023;1–10. https://doi.org/10.1017/cjn.2023.46. Available at: https://www.ncbi.nlm.nih.gov/pubmed/37113079.

61. Molina CA, Dibble CF, Lo SL, et al. Augmented reality-mediated stereotactic navigation for execution of en bloc lumbar spondylectomy osteotomies. J Neurosurg Spine 2021;1–6. https://doi.org/10.3171/2020.9.SPINE201219.

62. Hersh AM, Dedrickson T, Gong JH, et al. Neurosurgical utilization, charges, and reimbursement after the affordable care act: Trends from 2011 to 2019. Neurosurgery 2023;92(5):963–70. Available at: https://www.ncbi.nlm.nih.gov/pubmed/36700751.

63. Judy BF, Pennington Z, Botros D, et al. Spine image guidance and robotics: Exposure, education, training, and the learning curve. Int J Spine Surg 2021;15(s2):S28–37. Available at: https://search.proquest.com/docview/2584435541.

Advances in Implant Technologies for Spine Surgery

Shahab Aldin Sattari, MD[a,1], Yuanxuan Xia, MD[a,1], Tej D. Azad, MD, MS[a,b],
Chad A. Caraway, MS[a], Louis Chang, MD[a,*]

KEYWORDS

- Spine • Surgery • Implant • Prosthesis • Cage • Screw • Technology

KEY POINTS

- Three-dimensional (3D)-printed technology can create patient-specific prosthetics for spinal reconstruction and screw placement.
- Modifying interbody porosity and surface coating can improve osseous integration and reduce subsidence.
- Innovations in percutaneous pedicle screw systems have improved safety and efficiency.
- Carbon fiber-reinforced polyetheretherketone pedicle screws offer promising benefits in imaging evaluation and adjuvant treatment planning in spinal malignancies.
- Lumbar facet replacement devices offer a potential alternative to some spinal conditions traditionally considered for fusion surgeries.

INTRODUCTION

Spine implant materials continue to evolve to address the diverse needs of the multicompartment spine.[1] In only a few decades, a plethora of devices have emerged. The intervertebral disc can be replaced with interbody spacers or artificial discs, the vertebral body can be matched by cages for both structure and function, the stabilizing posterior elements can be reconstituted by the now-conventional pedicle screw and rod paradigm, just to name a few.[1] In this article, the authors discuss new developments in spine implants for both devices and materials. These advances in implant technology include three-dimensional (3D)-printed materials, expandable devices, specialized surface designs, pedicle screw techniques and construction, and novel facet replacements. The authors analyze these state-of-the-art technologies, their proposed uses, and consider future applications.

THREE-DIMENSIONAL-PRINTED TECHNOLOGY
Spine Prosthetics

Because 3D printing can be so personalized, multiple groups in recent years have evaluated its utility in complex reconstruction outcomes, particularly for en bloc resection of spinal tumors.[2–4] In patients undergoing total sacrectomies, 3D-printed prostheses have demonstrated more uniform stress distribution, lower peak stress, and better stability.[4] More recently, a small series reported on thoracolumbar tumor reconstructions using 3D-printed titanium alloy prosthetics and demonstrated proof of principle with reasonable clinical outcomes up to ~1 year follow-up.[2,3] These studies have shown a wide range of prosthesis subsidence but few cases of revision surgery. In direct comparisons between patients with 3D-printed titanium alloy and traditional titanium mesh cages, studies have noted

[a] Department of Neurosurgery, Johns Hopkins School of Medicine, Baltimore, Maryland, USA; [b] Department of Neurosurgery, Johns Hopkins Hospital, Johns Hopkins University School of Medicine, 1800 Orleans Street, 6007 Zayed Tower, Baltimore, MD 21287, USA
[1] These authors contributed equally.
* Corresponding author. Johns Hopkins School of Medicine, 10215 Fernwood Rd, Suite 412, Bethesda, MD 20817.
E-mail address: lchang10@jhmi.edu

Neurosurg Clin N Am 35 (2024) 217–227
https://doi.org/10.1016/j.nec.2023.11.003
1042-3680/24/© 2023 Elsevier Inc. All rights reserved.

non-inferiority in terms of fixation failure or subsidence and, in some cases, decreased rates of subsidence and back pain.[5,6]

SCREW APPLICATIONS

In addition to customized implants, 3D-printing has been used in preoperative planning for screw placement in terms of insertion point, path, length, and thickness of screws.[7] Such 3D-printed screw guide templates have helped further reduce instrumentation complications.[8,9]

This application has been used especially in deformity surgery to facilitate preoperative planning. In both adult degenerative scoliosis and adolescent idiopathic scoliosis, reports have detailed how preoperative 3D models have helped intraoperative screw trajectories with accurate placement within ~1 mm of optimal screw entry points and greater than 90% acceptable screw placement. Although such studies have been in small case series, comparisons to historical reports of misplaced freehand screws have been encouraging.[9,10]

Although the early findings suggest that 3D-printed patient-specific screw guides may improve the precision and safety of spinal procedures, more extensive and robust studies are required to elucidate their full potential in clinical practice.

Expandable Vertebral Body Replacement Cages

The anterior spinal column bears up to 75% of axial loading.[11] To optimize its reconstruction following corpectomy, expandable cages (**Fig. 1**A, B) have been applied in practice.[11–18]

The expandable feature of vertebral body replacement (VBR) cages has been studied for reducing subsidence, which complicates 80% of patients with anterior column reconstruction. In principle, maximizing end cap size may ameliorate loading stress and, thereby, decrease subsidence. Several reports have detailed the feasibility of using these expandable cages in a broad range of patient populations, from cervical to lumbar spine and for pathologies ranging from degenerative disease to malignancies, and confirmed improvement in standard clinical outcomes and low revision rates (eg, 1/40).[11,19] Radiographically, reports have shown greater than 90% fusion with these cages in both cervical and thoracolumbar locations, though subsidence rates up to 17% have been shown with 14-month follow-up.[13,14] As these studies had heterogeneous population, limited conclusions could be drawn. Nevertheless, the reports have indicated the feasibility of an expandable anchored titanium cage after anterior corpectomy.[15]

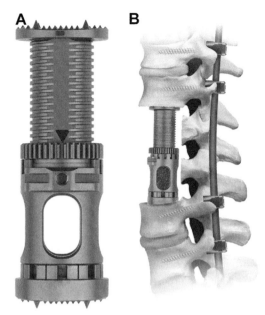

Fig. 1. Anterior view of expandable vertebral body replacement cage (A) and lateral view of Globus expandable VBR in thoracic spine (B).

One of the larger series on expandable VBR cages focused on traumatic thoracolumbar spinal fractures. After 2 years, 97.9% bony fusion and 4.2% total revision rates were reported.[16] A few other studies have also focused on specific patient populations including osteoporotic thoracolumbar fractures, post-traumatic kyphosis, and thoracolumbar metastases. In general, these reports have demonstrated good clinical outcomes, improved VAS scores, and kyphotic deformity parameters.[17–20] Interestingly, in those patients with osteoporotic thoracolumbar fractures, subgroup analyses suggested that Japanese Orthopedics Association scores were improved more in lumbar-only pathology than thoracolumbar pathology.[17] Further, in patients who underwent subaxial corpectomies, although there seemed to be low fusion rates (65.3% over 3 years), there were still improved rates of average VAS pain scores, neck disability index (NDI) scores, and Cobb angles.[20] Overall, though there are notable limitations, reports in recent years on expandable VBR cages have painted a favorable landscape for expandable VBR cages.

INTERBODY IMPLANT INNOVATIONS

Implant characteristics, including surface coating, chemistry, and topography including porosity and roughness, determine implant osteointegration and successful bony fusion. Therefore, evolving technologies have focused on optimizing all these features together in order to enhance fusion outcomes.[21]

EXPANDABLE INTERBODY IMPLANTS

As noted above with expandable VBR cages, devices that conform in situ offer several unique advantages in the surgical setting, namely that they require a smaller corridor for access while still providing for in vivo pathology correction. In TLIFs, Lin and colleagues' meta-analysis of expandable and static cages in 1440 patients showed higher anterior disc height and foraminal height, lower Oswestry disability index scores, and nonsignificant increase in posterior disc height and lordosis for the expandable cage group.[22] Conformational meshes have emerged as another type of expandable implants. They offer the additional advantage of integrating in accordance with the patient's anatomy. Stone and colleagues reported success with a radiolucent, porous polyester mesh pouch that is compatible with minimally invasive approaches offering multiple planes for graft–device interaction, promoting osteogenesis. This device was tested in a prospective, multicenter, single-arm FDA-approved investigational device exemption (IDE) trial. The study which enrolled 102 patients reported significant reduction in VAS back pain at 6 weeks and 24 months postoperatively. Similar reductions were noted in pain radiating to lower limbs and 99% fusion rates 2 years after surgery. No adverse events solely related to the implanted device were reported.[23] Of note, however, this particular study faced limitations such as lack of a control group and limited follow-up and needs to be validated by a future randomized study.

Porous Implants

Porous implants, by virtue of their construction and osteointegration, result in a more mechanically stable column and lower risk of fusion failure. Increased bone–device interface results in lower rates of disc subsidence and early bone fusion, as proven in canine[24] and ovine models under standardized stress settings.[25] Fogel and colleagues evaluated the potential effects of porous bodies (lattice vs solid) and endplates (microporous vs smooth) on cage stiffness and subsidence in an ovine interbody fusion model. There were 16.7% and 16.6% reduction in cage stiffness by using porous body lattice and microporous endplate, indicating that body lattice and microporous endplates characteristic can enhance early fusion through cage stiffness and stress shielding reduction. Furthermore, porous titanium cage showed the lowest stiffness and block stiffness (**Fig. 2**).

Owing to stiffness reduction, and hence optimized osteointegration and potential diminished subsidence, they hypothesized that porous titanium cage may be a viable option in clinical settings.[25] In terms of subsidence, Kraftt and colleagues showed that 3D-printed porous titanium intervertebral cages in lateral interbody fusions showed a subsidence rate of 6.7%, though all were clinically irrelevant and did not require revision operation.[26] Porous polyetheretherketone (PEEK) implants have been reported in multilevel anterior cervical discectomy and fusions procedures (**Fig. 3**), with data suggesting good clinical outcomes. Out of 33 patients with ≥3-level anterior cervical discectomy and fusion (ACDFs), two patients developed cage subsidence (6.1%) and one patient had pseudoarthrosis (3%), though overall successful fusion rate was recorded at 97%, which supersedes established rates for complex cohorts.[27]

Surface-Coated Technologies

Antimicrobial-coated orthopedic implants have already proven to be efficacious and safe in clinical use.[28] Silver (Ag), copper (Cu), and iodine (I) are candidates for coated implants, with delivery also possible through a variety of techniques.[29] Application in spinal surgery with the use of silver and hydroxyapatite surface-coated lumbar interbody cage was recently reported by Morimoto and colleagues which showed promising results.[30] In another small study comparing titanium-coated versus uncoated PEEK cage in single-level

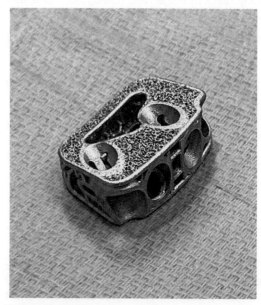

Fig. 2. Nuvasive anterior lumbar interbody fusion (ALIF) Modulus implant.

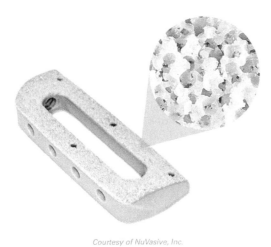

Courtesy of NuVasive, Inc.

Fig. 3. Nuvasive porous PEEK Cohere extreme lateral interbody fusion (XLIF) implant. (*Courtesy of* NuVasive.)

posterior lumbar interbody fusion, 3-month fusion rates were 88% and quantified vertebral cancellous condensation, as an index of bone ingrowth, were significantly greater in titanium-coated cages, suggesting titanium coatings may promote solid fusion and enhance the outcomes of interbody fusions.[31]

SCREW INNOVATIONS
Minimally Invasive Spine Surgery

Minimally invasive spine surgery (MISS) has been defined by key technologies, notably percutaneous pedicle screw systems. This technique has significantly changed since its initial description in the early 1980s by Magerl and colleagues,[32] now with a currently established insertion technique of:[33]

1. X-ray imaging for localization (eg, fluoroscopy or CT scan)
2. Skin incision and blunt dissection of fascia
3. Jamshidi needle to dock at screw insertion site
4. Kirschner (K)-wire placement
5. Repeat X-ray imaging for confirmation of screw insertion site
6. Breach cortical bone using the K-wire as a guide (ie, with a cannulated awl)
7. Successive dilators
8. Tunneling or "tapping" through a pedicle
9. Cannulated screw placement over the K-wire
10. Repeat X-ray imaging for final screw confirmation

Recently, fourth-generation percutaneous pedicle screw systems have streamlined the screw insertion process further. Systems like the VIPER PRIME (DePuy Synthes Spine, Raynham, MA, USA) (**Fig.** 4A–I),[34] Voyager ATMAS (Medtronic,

Memphis, TN, USA), and RELINE ONE (NuVasive, San Diego, CA, USA) (**Fig.** 5A–C) consolidate many of the above steps into a single instrument pass while using intraoperative navigation. These systems remove the need for Jamshidi needles, K-wires, dilators, tapping of cancellous bone, or multiple radiation exposures. Ultimately, these "all-in-one" instruments can abbreviate a screw insertion process to.

1. Intraoperative scan for navigation
2. Skin incision
3. Navigated placement of screwdriver system to desired insertion point
4. Screw insertion
5. Repeat intraoperative scan for hardware placement confirmation (optional)

Although the fourth-generation systems achieve this integrated approach with different mechanisms, the common factor is a single device that allows for maneuvering a screw to a desired insertion point, breaching cortical bone, and tunneling through a pedicle. Previously, each of these steps involved an exchange between the operator and assistant. However, with all-in-one instruments, a significant amount of time is saved per screw; the VIPER PRIME[35] claims a 60% reduction in screw insertion time. This has been corroborated by multiple groups and a significant reduction in operative time has been confirmed across similar systems, although studies define differently what is the time required for screw insertion.[36–38] Beyond saving time, removing the K-wire also reduces risks as it has been implicated in various complications related to displacement or bending (eg, cerebral spinal fluid [CSF] leak and retroperitoneal hematoma).[39]

Biomechanical data on the all-in-one screw systems, although sparse, have been promising in demonstrating at least non-inferiority. Pereira and colleagues showed no significant difference in pullout forces, fixation stiffness, or screw displacement necessary for pullout in cadaveric spines using both new and conventional systems.[40] Early clinical reports have also shown minimal complication rates. Misplacement and breach of screws have been reported at ~10%, which is comparable to current minimally-invasive spine surgery (MISS) techniques of 6% to 23% and remains improved compared with the upward of 39% breach rates in a traditional open approach.[37,38]

Carbon Fiber-Reinforced Polyetheretherketone

Modern titanium instruments are strong fixation devices that reliably immobilize the spine. However, a

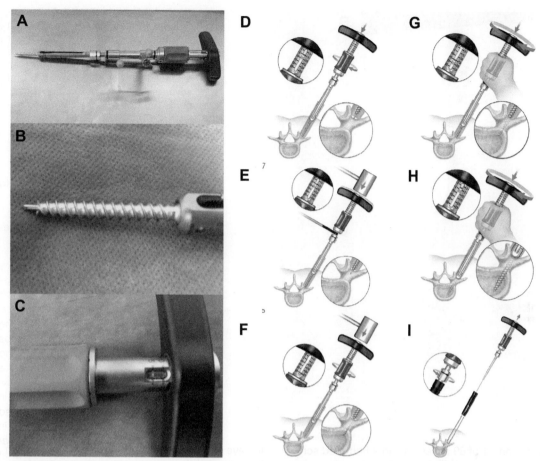

Fig. 4. (*A*) VIPER PRIME screw inserter assembled with a navigation tower. (*B*) At baseline, the stylet rests ~3 mm past the screw tip. (*C*) Expanded view of the handle with red stylet depth line. Screw insertion involves (*D*) docking at desired location and turning red handle clockwise to extend stylet past the screw tip as you (*E*) mallet the stylet into bone and through pedicle. (*F*) The depth gauge (expanded view) indicates how far the stylet is past the screw tip. (*G*) Insert screw by holding the red stylet handle still and turning the T-handle. (*H*) The red line decreases toward its baseline as the screw advances. (*I*) Turn green knob to disengage the inserter assembly from the screw.

persistent problem has been the imaging artifact caused by the metal, which restricts postoperative MRI and CT evaluation.[41] The thermoplastic polymer PEEK helped address this problem as PEEK systems are radiolucent and have been commonly used in cervical spine surgery.[42] However, their semirigid design limits long-term fusion because they permit continued micromovements.[43] In recent years, integrating carbon fiber into the PEEK matrix has generated a rigid and radiolucent material for screw designs and instrumentation.

In biomechanical studies, carbon fiber-reinforced PEEK (CFR PEEK) is equivalent to titanium constructs in both biocompatibility and biomechanical properties.[41] Studies across CFR PEEK systems have shown similar properties compared with known titanium constructs for mean bending yield load, fatigue from cyclic axial compression, and

pullout strength.[44,45] The benefits of CFR PEEK have mostly focused on their potential in oncology patients. Presumably, radiolucent constructs (**Fig. 6**A–C) facilitate imaging evaluation and increased accuracy for radiotherapy planning in the short term and more easily detect local recurrence in the long term. However, few studies have objectively evaluated the benefits of CFR PEEK in postoperative radiation planning. Müller and colleagues compared radiation planning accuracy on five patients with CFR PEEK screws and five with standard titanium alloy screws and found that CFR PEEK allowed for a reduced standard deviation in target volume measurements.[46] By extension, CFR PEEK systems allowed for more accurate and precise postoperative radiation planning.

Intraoperatively, retrospective series show low complications with CFR PEEK including 1 of 34

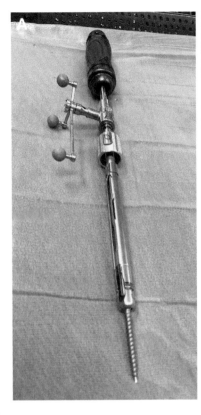
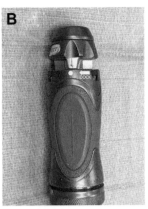
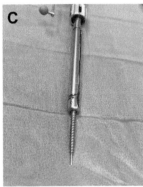

Fig. 5. (*A*) Nuvasive RELINE ONE all-in-one cannulated pedicle screws with extended tabs. The awl-tipped vector enables docking and breaching of cortical bone. The vector is then extended further (*B*) by rotation and advancement of the handle cap to guide the screw in its determined trajectory (*C*).

cases and 1 of 69 cases having a fractured screw during insertion.[47,48] A recent systematic review on CFR PEEK for primary and metastatic spine tumor patients showed similar operative outcomes compared with titanium implants.[49] Pedicle screw fractures occurred in 1.7% of CFR PEEK cases and 2.4% of titanium constructs. Reoperation occurred in 5.7% of CFR PEEK systems and 4.8% of titanium constructs. Multiple groups are actively collecting long-term oncologic outcomes, but current limited cumulative data have shown an overall local recurrence rate of 13.0% more than 13.5 months average follow-up.

Despite its promise, common limitations to CFR PEEK systems have been recognized.[48] Current products cannot be bent to suit individual anatomy intraoperatively and available pre-bent options may not suit every individual case. Ultimately, it is unclear whether the presumed increase in postoperative imaging accuracy and higher chance of detecting local recurrence generates a significant clinical impact on oncology patient outcomes. Recent commentary on CFR PEEK systems pointed out how the continued evolution of targeted therapies and immunotherapies in oncology are what will really affect these patients' outcomes.[50] However, for spine tumors that continue to have limited systemic options and still rely on en bloc surgical therapy, such as primary chordoma and chondrosarcoma tumors, CFR PEEK systems may substantially impact their postoperative course. In part due to this unclear effect on outcomes and also from the considerable increase in costs, CFR PEEK systems have not yet been widely adopted.

Facet Replacement Devices

Lumbar facet arthroplasty (LFA), using facet replacement devices (FRD), has been proposed as a method for achieving dynamic spinal stabilization. Although several FRD systems have emerged for LFA, including the Anatomic Facet Replacement System (Facet Solutions Inc, acquired by Globus Medical) and the Total Facet Arthroplasty System (TFAS) (Archus Orthopedics, acquired by Globus Medical), the Total Posterior Spine System (TOPS) (Premia Spine) is the only such device with FDA approval thus far (FDA PMA number P220002).[51]

The TOPS consists of a motion implant and four pedicle screws (**Fig. 7**A, B). The motion implant is defined as two titanium endplates connected by a polyurethane chamber. This chamber houses titanium and polycarbonate urethane articulating

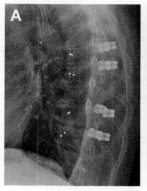 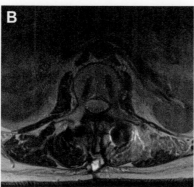 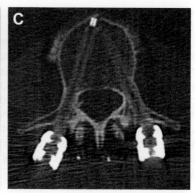

Fig. 6. (A) Sagittal X-ray of thoracolumbar CFR PEEK instrumentation (icotec ag, Altstätten, Switzerland) demonstrating their radiolucent screw shafts. Postoperative MRI (B) and CT (C) demonstrating reduced imaging artifact. (Image B, *Courtesy of* prof. Ehab Shiban, department of neurosurgery, university hospital of Augsburg, Germany.)

components and a woven PEEK ribbon. Following a standard midline posterior approach, four pedicle screws are placed at the cranial and caudal levels, followed by placement of the TOPS motion implant.[52] Coric and colleagues published findings from the prospective, randomized TOPS FDA IDE trial for one-level symptomatic lumbar stenosis with grade 1 degenerative spondylolisthesis. A greater percentage of patients in the TOPS group (85%) met a composite outcome at 24 months than in the transforaminal lumbar interbody fusion (TLIF) group (64%).[53] This work followed initial results from the investigational arm reported by Pinter and colleagues.[54] An important limitation of this work is the relatively short follow-up for the outcome of adjacent segment disease. Small, prospective studies suggest clinical improvement, maintained range of motion, and low rates of reoperation at 5[55] and 11 years.[56]

The Anatomic Facet Replacement System (AFRS) also uses traditional pedicle screw fixation, which is then connected by a cross-link at the caudal aspect of the construct. AFRS consists of PEEK, titanium alloys, cobalt chromium alloy, commercially pure titanium, and hydroxyapatite.[57] An FDA IDE trial (NCT00401518) comparing AFRS

with posterior lumbar fusion (PLF) for spinal stenosis was initiated in 2006 and completed in 2017, though the final results have not been published. Preliminary trial results suggest that similar clinical improvements and reoperation rates at between AFRS and PLF at 2 and 4 years.[58] Of note, there has been a case report (*N* = 2) describing cobalt allergies (a key component of the implant "metal on metal" motion preservation design) with local tissue reaction and return of neurologic symptoms requiring revision to traditional titanium PLF.[59]

The TFAS is composed of a rostral "L"-shaped stems anchored to a caudal motion-preserving system. TFAS is anchored via straight stems passing into the vertebral body via a traditional pedicle screw trajectory. The straight stems are secured using polymethyl methacrylate cement.[60,61] Clinical evidence for TFAS is limited. A small series (*N* = 14) was reported in 2014 with a mean follow-up of 3.7 years and revealed consistent improvement in clinical outcomes and preserved motion on dynamic radiographs.[62] An FDA IDE trial (NCT00418197) was initiated in 2005 to compare TFAS with PLF, but not completed. Preliminary results (TFAS, *N* = 96; PLF, *N* = 8) suggest that the device may yield comparable clinical improvements compared with PLF.[63] Importantly, a case

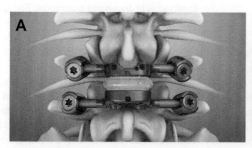 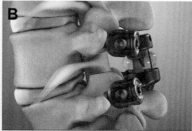

Fig. 7. Anterior-posterior (A) and lateral (B) illustrations of Total Posterior Spine System.

report (N = 2) described breakage of the stems requiring revision interbody fusion.[64]

Although FRDs offer a motion-preserving option to traditional fusion for degenerative spinal pathology, further research is required. Initial clinical results suggest that these devices can provide clinical improvements in pain and disability, though it is difficult to determine if improvements are attributable to decompression of neural elements. Long-term studies are required to thoroughly understand the impact of FRDs on adjacent segment disease.

SUMMARY

Spine implants are becoming increasingly diversified. Taking inspiration from other industries, 3D modeling of the spinal column has helped meet the custom needs of individual patients as both en bloc replacements and pedicle screw designs. Intraoperative tailoring of devices, a common need in the operating room, has led to expandable versions of cages and interbody spacers. The implant surface has been scrutinized as collaborations with other surgical fields have found certain compounds with antimicrobial and fusion-promoting properties. These partnerships have also changed the composition of implants themselves, with carbon-fiber reinforced compounds representing a hopeful addition to the spine oncology arsenal. Techniques with existing implants have also advanced, with minimally invasive "all-in-one" pedicle screws streamlining instrumentation steps in the operating room. Finally, new treatment paradigms continue to emerge, including facet replacement devices that may help treat degenerative spine pathology in a new light.

DISCLOSURE

Louis Chang: Nuvasive consultant educator, sponsored principal investigator.

ACKNOWLEDGMENT

The authors would like to thank Dr Angad Grewal for his help in this project.

REFERENCES

1. Martz EO, Goel VK, Pope MH, et al. Materials and design of spinal implants–a review. J Biomed Mater Res 1997;38(3):267–88.
2. Girolami M, Boriani S, Bandiera S, et al. Biomimetic 3D-printed custom-made prosthesis for anterior column reconstruction in the thoracolumbar spine: a tailored option following en bloc resection for spinal tumors : Preliminary results on a case-series of 13 patients. Eur spine J Off Publ Eur Spine Soc Eur Spinal Deform Soc Eur Sect Cerv Spine Res Soc 2018; 27(12):3073–83.
3. Tang X, Yang Y, Zang J, et al. Preliminary Results of a 3D-Printed Modular Vertebral Prosthesis for Anterior Column Reconstruction after Multilevel Thoracolumbar Total En Bloc Spondylectomy. Orthop Surg 2021;13(3):949–57. https://doi.org/10.1111/os. 12975.
4. Huang S, Ji T, Guo W. Biomechanical comparison of a 3D-printed sacrum prosthesis versus rod-screw systems for reconstruction after total sacrectomy: A finite element analysis. Clin Biomech 2019;70: 203–8. https://doi.org/10.1016/j.clinbiomech.2019. 10.019.
5. Chen Z, Lü G, Wang X, et al. Is 3D-printed prosthesis stable and economic enough for anterior spinal column reconstruction after spinal tumor resection? A retrospective comparative study between 3D-printed off-the-shelf prosthesis and titanium mesh cage. Eur spine J Off Publ Eur Spine Soc Eur Spinal Deform Soc Eur Sect Cerv Spine Res Soc 2023;32(1):261–70. https://doi.org/10. 1007/s00586-022-07480-9.
6. Dong C, Wei H, Zhu Y, et al. Application of Titanium Alloy 3D-Printed Artificial Vertebral Body for Stage III Kümmell's Disease Complicated by Neurological Deficits. Clin Interv Aging 2020;15:2265–76. https://doi.org/10.2147/CIA.S283809.
7. Tong Y, Kaplan DJ, Spivak JM, et al. Three-dimensional printing in spine surgery: a review of current applications. Spine J 2020;20(6):833–46. https:// doi.org/10.1016/j.spinee.2019.11.004.
8. Senkoylu A, Cetinkaya M, Daldal I, et al. Personalized Three-Dimensional Printing Pedicle Screw Guide Innovation for the Surgical Management of Patients with Adolescent Idiopathic Scoliosis. World Neurosurg 2020;144:e513–22. https://doi.org/10. 1016/j.wneu.2020.08.212.
9. Matsukawa K, Abe Y, Mobbs RJ. Novel Technique for Sacral-Alar-Iliac Screw Placement Using Three-Dimensional Patient-Specific Template Guide. Spine Surg Relat Res 2021;5(6):418–24. https://doi.org/10. 22603/ssrr.2020-0221.
10. Modi HN, Suh SW, Fernandez H, et al. Accuracy and safety of pedicle screw placement in neuromuscular scoliosis with free-hand technique. Eur spine J Off Publ Eur Spine Soc Eur Spinal Deform Soc Eur Sect Cerv Spine Res Soc 2008;17(12):1686–96. https://doi.org/10.1007/s00586-008-0795-6.
11. Stinchfield T, Vadapalli S, Pennington Z, et al. Improvement in vertebral endplate engagement following anterior column reconstruction using a novel expandable cage with self-adjusting, multiaxial end cap. J Clin Neurosci Off J Neurosurg Soc Australas 2019;67:249–54. https://doi.org/10. 1016/j.jocn.2019.06.017.

12. Cappelletto B, Giorgiutti F, Balsano M. Evaluation of the effectiveness of expandable cages for reconstruction of the anterior column of the spine. J Orthop Surg 2020;28(1). https://doi.org/10.1177/2309499019900472. 2309499019900472.

13. Deml MC, Mazuret Sepulveda CA, Albers CE, et al. Anterior column reconstruction of the thoracolumbar spine with a new modular PEEK vertebral body replacement device: retrospective clinical and radiologic cohort analysis of 48 cases with 1.7-years follow-up. Eur spine J Off Publ Eur Spine Soc Eur Spinal Deform Soc Eur Sect Cerv Spine Res Soc 2020;29(12):3194–202. https://doi.org/10.1007/s00586-020-06464-x.

14. Pojskic M, Saß B, Nimsky C, et al. Application of an Expandable Cage for Reconstruction of the Cervical Spine in a Consecutive Series of Eighty-Six Patients. Medicina (Kaunas). 2020;56(12). https://doi.org/10.3390/medicina56120642.

15. Yusupov N, Siller S, Hofereiter J, et al. Vertebral Body Replacement With an Anchored Expandable Titanium Cage in the Cervical Spine: A Clinical and Radiological Evaluation. Oper Neurosurg (Hagerstown, Md) 2020;20(1):109–18. https://doi.org/10.1093/ons/opaa296.

16. Lang S, Neumann C, Schwaiger C, et al. Radiological and mid- to long-term patient-reported outcome after stabilization of traumatic thoraco-lumbar spinal fractures using an expandable vertebral body replacement implant. BMC Muscoskel Disord 2021;22(1):744. https://doi.org/10.1186/s12891-021-04585-y.

17. Terai H, Takahashi S, Yasuda H, et al. Differences in surgical outcome after anterior corpectomy and reconstruction with an expandable cage with rectangular footplates between thoracolumbar and lumbar osteoporotic vertebral fracture. North Am Spine Soc J 2021;6:100071. https://doi.org/10.1016/j.xnsj.2021.100071.

18. Kang D, Lewis SJ, Kim D-H. Clinical Efficacy and Safety of Controlled Distraction-Compression Technique Using Expandable Titanium Cage in Correction of Posttraumatic Kyphosis. J Korean Neurosurg Soc 2022;65(1):84–95. https://doi.org/10.3340/jkns.2021.0147.

19. Ulu MO, Akgun MY, Alizada O, et al. Posterior-only approach in patients with poor general condition and spinal metastatic vertebral fracture. Neurocir 2023. https://doi.org/10.1016/j.neucie.2022.10.002. English Ed. Published online March.

20. Byvaltsev VA, Kalinin AA, Belykh EG, et al. Clinical and radiological outcomes of one-level cervical corpectomy with an expandable cage for three-column uncomplicated subaxial type «B» injures: a multicenter retrospective study. Eur spine J Off Publ Eur Spine Soc Eur Spinal Deform Soc Eur Sect Cerv Spine Res Soc 2023;32(5):1644–54. https://doi.org/10.1007/s00586-023-07648-x.

21. Chan JL, Bae HW, Harrison Farber S, et al. Evolution of Bioactive Implants in Lateral Interbody Fusion. Int J spine Surg 2022;16(S1):S61–8. https://doi.org/10.14444/8237.

22. Lin G-X, Kim J-S, Kotheeranurak V, et al. Does the application of expandable cages in TLIF provide improved clinical and radiological results compared to static cages? A meta-analysis. Front Surg 2022;9:949938. https://doi.org/10.3389/fsurg.2022.949938.

23. Chi JH, Nunley PD, Huang KT, et al. Two-Year Outcomes From a Prospective Multicenter Investigation Device Trial of a Novel Conformal Mesh Interbody Fusion Device. Int J spine Surg 2021;15(6):1103–14. https://doi.org/10.14444/8169.

24. Takemoto M, Fujibayashi S, Neo M, et al. A porous bioactive titanium implant for spinal interbody fusion: an experimental study using a canine model. J Neurosurg Spine 2007;7(4):435–43. https://doi.org/10.3171/SPI-07/10/435.

25. Fogel G, Martin N, Lynch K, et al. Subsidence and fusion performance of a 3D-printed porous interbody cage with stress-optimized body lattice and microporous endplates - a comprehensive mechanical and biological analysis. Spine J 2022;22(6):1028–37. https://doi.org/10.1016/j.spinee.2022.01.003.

26. Krafft PR, Osburn B, Vivas AC, et al. Novel Titanium Cages for Minimally Invasive Lateral Lumbar Interbody Fusion: First Assessment of Subsidence. Spine Surg Relat Res 2020;4(2):171–7. https://doi.org/10.22603/ssrr.2019-0089.

27. Basques BA, Gomez G, Padovano A, et al. Porous Polyetheretherketone Interbody Cages for Anterior Cervical Discectomy and Fusion at 3 or More Levels: Clinical and Radiographic Outcomes. Int J spine Surg 2023;17(2):215–21. https://doi.org/10.14444/8410.

28. Savvidou OD, Kaspiris A, Trikoupis I, et al. Efficacy of antimicrobial coated orthopaedic implants on the prevention of periprosthetic infections: a systematic review and meta-analysis. J bone Jt Infect 2020;5(4):212–22. https://doi.org/10.7150/jbji.44839.

29. Morimoto T, Hirata H, Eto S, et al. Development of Silver-Containing Hydroxyapatite-Coated Antimicrobial Implants for Orthopaedic and Spinal Surgery. Medicina (Kaunas). 2022;58(4). https://doi.org/10.3390/medicina58040519.

30. Morimoto T, Tsukamoto M, Aita K, et al. First clinical experience with posterior lumbar interbody fusion using a thermal-sprayed silver-containing hydroxyapatite-coated cage. J Orthop Surg Res 2023;18(1):392. https://doi.org/10.1186/s13018-023-03882-7.

31. Kashii M, Kitaguchi K, Makino T, et al. Comparison in the same intervertebral space between titanium-coated and uncoated PEEK cages in lumbar interbody fusion surgery. J Orthop Sci Off J Japanese Orthop Assoc 2020;25(4):565–70. https://doi.org/10.1016/j.jos.2019.07.004.

32. Magerl FP. Stabilization of the lower thoracic and lumbar spine with external skeletal fixation. Clin Orthop Relat Res 1984;189:125–41.

33. Ishii K, Funao H, Isogai N, et al. The History and Development of the Percutaneous Pedicle Screw (PPS) System. Medicina (Kaunas). 2022;58(8). https://doi.org/10.3390/medicina58081064.

34. Chang L, Kimaz S, Wipplinger C, et al. Posterior thoracic and lumbar instrumentation. In: Winn HR, editor. Youmans & Winn's Neurological Surgery, 8/e. Philadelphia: Elsevier; 2023. Video 362.1.

35. VIPER PRIME TM System Cadaver Time Study. DePuy Synthes White Paper. August 24, 2017. Accessed July 8, 2023.

36. Kojima A, Aihara T, Urushibara M, et al. Safety and Efficacy of All-In-One Percutaneous Pedicle Screw System. Glob spine J 2023;13(4):970–6. https://doi.org/10.1177/21925682211011440.

37. Schmidt FA, Lekuya HM, Kirnaz S, et al. Novel MIS 3D NAV Single Step Pedicle Screw System (SSPSS): Workflow, Accuracy and Initial Clinical Experience. Glob spine J 2022;12(6):1098–108. https://doi.org/10.1177/2192568220976393.

38. Sadrameli SS, Jafrani R, Staub BN, et al. Minimally Invasive, Stereotactic, Wireless, Percutaneous Pedicle Screw Placement in the Lumbar Spine: Accuracy Rates With 182 Consecutive Screws. Int J spine Surg 2018;12(6):650–8. https://doi.org/10.14444/5081.

39. Mobbs RJ, Raley DA. Complications with K-wire insertion for percutaneous pedicle screws. J Spinal Disord Tech 2014;27(7):390–4. https://doi.org/10.1097/BSD.0b013e3182999380.

40. de Andrada Pereira B, O'Neill LK, Sawa AGU, et al. Biomechanical Assessment of a Novel Sharp-Tipped Screw for 1-Step Minimally Invasive Pedicle Screw Placement Under Navigation. Int J spine Surg 2023. https://doi.org/10.14444/8470.

41. Ponnappan RK, Serhan H, Zarda B, et al. Biomechanical evaluation and comparison of polyetheretherketone rod system to traditional titanium rod fixation. Spine J 2009;9(3):263–7. https://doi.org/10.1016/j.spinee.2008.08.002.

42. Kersten RFMR, van Gaalen SM, de Gast A, et al. Polyetheretherketone (PEEK) cages in cervical applications: a systematic review. Spine J 2015;15(6):1446–60. https://doi.org/10.1016/j.spinee.2013.08.030.

43. Galbusera F, Bellini CM, Anasetti F, et al. Rigid and flexible spinal stabilization devices: a biomechanical comparison. Med Eng Phys 2011;33(4):490–6. https://doi.org/10.1016/j.medengphy.2010.11.018.

44. Uri O, Folman Y, Laufer G, et al. A Novel Spine Fixation System Made Entirely of Carbon-Fiber-Reinforced PEEK Composite: An In Vitro Mechanical Evaluation. Adv Orthop 2020;2020:4796136. https://doi.org/10.1155/2020/4796136.

45. Oikonomidis S, Greven J, Bredow J, et al. Biomechanical effects of posterior pedicle screw-based instrumentation using titanium versus carbon fiber reinforced PEEK in an osteoporotic spine human cadaver model. Clin Biomech 2020;80:105153. https://doi.org/10.1016/j.clinbiomech.2020.105153.

46. Müller BS, Ryang Y-M, Oechsner M, et al. The dosimetric impact of stabilizing spinal implants in radiotherapy treatment planning with protons and photons: standard titanium alloy vs. radiolucent carbon-fiber-reinforced PEEK systems. J Appl Clin Med Phys 2020;21(8):6–14. https://doi.org/10.1002/acm2.12905.

47. Boriani S, Tedesco G, Ming L, et al. Carbon-fiber-reinforced PEEK fixation system in the treatment of spine tumors: a preliminary report. Eur spine J Off Publ Eur Spine Soc Eur Spinal Deform Soc Eur Sect Cerv Spine Res Soc 2018;27(4):874–81. https://doi.org/10.1007/s00586-017-5258-5.

48. Alvarez-Breckenridge C, de Almeida R, Haider A, et al. Carbon Fiber-Reinforced Polyetheretherketone Spinal Implants for Treatment of Spinal Tumors: Perceived Advantages and Limitations. Neurospine 2023;20(1):317–26. https://doi.org/10.14245/ns.2244920.460.

49. Khan HA, Ber R, Neifert SN, et al. Carbon fiber-reinforced PEEK spinal implants for primary and metastatic spine tumors: a systematic review on implant complications and radiotherapy benefits. J Neurosurg Spine 2023;1–14. https://doi.org/10.3171/2023.5.SPINE23106.

50. Chi JH. Commentary on "Carbon Fiber-Reinforced Polyetheretherketone Spinal Implants for Treatment of Spinal Tumors: Perceived Advantages and Limitations". Neurospine 2023;20(1):327–8. https://doi.org/10.14245/ns.2346314.157.

51. Gu BJ, Blue R, Yoon J, et al. Posterior Lumbar Facet Replacement and Arthroplasty. Neurosurg Clin N Am 2021;32(4):521–6. https://doi.org/10.1016/j.nec.2021.05.011.

52. McAfee P, Khoo LT, Pimenta L, et al. Treatment of lumbar spinal stenosis with a total posterior arthroplasty prosthesis: implant description, surgical technique, and a prospective report on 29 patients. Neurosurg Focus 2007;22(1):E13. https://doi.org/10.3171/foc.2007.22.1.13.

53. Coric D, Nassr A, Kim PK, et al. Prospective, randomized controlled multicenter study of posterior lumbar facet arthroplasty for the treatment of spondylolisthesis. J Neurosurg Spine 2023;38(1):115–25. https://doi.org/10.3171/2022.7.SPINE22536.

54. Pinter ZW, Freedman BA, Nassr A, et al. A Prospective Study of Lumbar Facet Arthroplasty in the Treatment of Degenerative Spondylolisthesis and Stenosis: Results from the Total Posterior Spine System (TOPS) IDE Study. Clin spine Surg 2023;36(2):E59–69. https://doi.org/10.1097/BSD.0000000000001365.

55. Haleem S, Ahmed A, Ganesan S, et al. Mean 5-Year Follow-Up Results of a Facet Replacement Device in the Treatment of Lumbar Spinal Stenosis and Degenerative Spondylolisthesis. World Neurosurg 2021;152:e645–51. https://doi.org/10.1016/j.wneu.2021.06.045.

56. Smorgick Y, Mirovsky Y, Floman Y, et al. Long-term results for total lumbar facet joint replacement in the management of lumbar degenerative spondylolisthesis. J Neurosurg Spine 2019;1–6. https://doi.org/10.3171/2019.7.SPINE19150.

57. Goel VK, Mehta A, Jangra J, et al. Anatomic Facet Replacement System (AFRS) Restoration of Lumbar Segment Mechanics to Intact: A Finite Element Study and In Vitro Cadaver Investigation. SAS J 2007;1(1):46–54. https://doi.org/10.1016/SASJ-2006-0010-RR.

58. Myer J, Youssef JA, Rahn KA, et al. ACADIA® facet replacement system IDE study: preliminary outcomes at two-and four-years postoperative. Spine J 2014;14(11):S160–1.

59. Goodwin ML, Spiker WR, Brodke DS, et al. Failure of facet replacement system with metal-on-metal bearing surface and subsequent discovery of cobalt allergy: report of 2 cases. J Neurosurg Spine 2018;29(1):81–4. https://doi.org/10.3171/2017.10.SPINE17862.

60. Phillips FM, Tzermiadianos MN, Voronov LI, et al. Effect of the Total Facet Arthroplasty System after complete laminectomy-facetectomy on the biomechanics of implanted and adjacent segments. Spine J 2009;9(1):96–102. https://doi.org/10.1016/j.spinee.2008.01.010.

61. Sjovold SG, Zhu Q, Bowden A, et al. Biomechanical evaluation of the Total Facet Arthroplasty System® (TFAS®): loading as compared to a rigid posterior instrumentation system. Eur spine J Off Publ Eur Spine Soc Eur Spinal Deform Soc Eur Sect Cerv Spine Res Soc 2012;21(8):1660–73. https://doi.org/10.1007/s00586-012-2253-8.

62. Vermesan D, Prejbeanu R, Daliborca CV, et al. A new device used in the restoration of kinematics after total facet arthroplasty. Med Devices (Auckl) 2014;7:157–63. https://doi.org/10.2147/MDER.S60945.

63. Sachs B, Webb S, Brown C, et al. The Total Facet Arthroplasty System®(TFAS®) in the Treatment of Degenerative Lumbar Spinal Stenosis: Midterm Results of US IDE Trial with Longest Follow-Up of 24-Months. Spine J 2008;8(5):60S–1S, 119.

64. Palmer DK, Inceoglu S, Cheng WK. Stem fracture after total facet replacement in the lumbar spine: a report of two cases and review of the literature. Spine J 2011;11(7):e15–9. https://doi.org/10.1016/j.spinee.2011.06.002.

Smart Spine Implants

Rory K.J. Murphy, MD[1]

KEYWORDS

- Sensors • Smart spine implants • Stimulation • Wireless

KEY POINTS

- Smart spine implants promise to stimulate healing and provide objective information about postoperative healing.
- The therapeutic potential of implants includes the ability to stimulate bone growth.
- Objective data during implantation and continuous postoperative data transfer combined with machine learning analysis could change practice patterns.
- Widespread adoption of smart spine implants may vary depending on cost and regulatory constraints.

INTRODUCTION/HISTORY/DEFINITIONS/BACKGROUND

Smart spine implants promise to stimulate healing and provide objective information about healing progression. The ability of smart spine implants to accelerate healing and provide objective data could help guide postoperative care, foster better outcomes, and reduce complications.[1]

Pacemakers and other cardiac devices have had data-transmission capabilities for years. They can track battery life and features of the device itself, as well as signs of new heart problems in the patient, such as arrhythmia. Smart knee replacement implants, introduced in 2021, are now in widespread clinical use.[2,3] Built-in sensors wirelessly transmit data to orthopedic surgeons. In addition, a sensor-equipped surgical trauma plate was recently developed that continuously and objectively monitors bone healing progression (Fracture Monitor; AO Foundation).[4] It includes an implantable data logger attached to a standard bone plate and a smartphone application that wirelessly connects with the data logger, downloading the information. A central Web server collects and stores data from the patient's smartphone for visualization.

Spinal implants will emulate current cardiology and orthopedic implants. Spine implants' small size and mechanical strength requirements present a packaging challenge to adding these smart capabilities. To date, these constraints have hindered the practical clinical use of smart spinal implants. However, new miniaturized wireless technology can fit into standard intervertebral spacers, plates, and pedicle screws. An increased number of smart implants will soon become available to help patients.

New smart spine implants that wirelessly transmit data to surgeons will personalize patient care. Data collected over months and years and analyzed with machine learning will allow spine surgeons to help patients reach their milestones. If performance data are concerning, a spine surgeon can intervene to order appropriate imaging or changes in treatment. This technology will enable remote checkups from home, which will be easier for patients and a more efficient use of health care resources.

Department of Neurosurgery, Barrow Neurological Institute, Neuroscience Publications, St. Joseph's Hospital and Medical Center, 350 West Thomas Road, Phoenix, AZ 85013, USA
[1] Present address: c/o Neuroscience Publications, Barrow Neurological Institute, St. Joseph's Hospital and Medical Center, 350 W. Thomas Rd, Phoenix, AZ 85013, USA
E-mail address: Neuropub@barrowneuro.org

Neurosurg Clin N Am 35 (2024) 229–234
https://doi.org/10.1016/j.nec.2023.11.002

Closed-loop control is a method used in many types of processes. It refers to a system that can automatically adjust process inputs to yield a desired process output. A common example is a home's air conditioning system, which automatically monitors air temperature and adjusts the system to yield the desired air temperature. This simple idea is harnessed in some medical devices, such as pacemakers, but has not yet been used in orthopedic implants. Closed-loop treatment will be enabled by smart spine implants, combining therapeutics (electrical stimulation of bone growth) directly linked to diagnostics (impedance measurements to detect new bone growth). Bone growth will be monitored remotely through a cloud-connected system. If data suggest poor healing, therapy can be activated through the implant. Today, all the decisions regarding the type of implant, allograft, autograft, and recombinant bone morphogenetic protein must be made before surgery. Smart implants may be used initially in monitoring-only mode, then remotely activated to provide treatment if required.

This article discusses early smart spine implants, current smart spine implants and their enabling technology, and future directions.

SMART SPINAL IMPLANTS PAST, PRESENT, AND FUTURE

One of the early applications of smart spine implants was the translation of strain gauges onto spinal rods for in vivo use. In 1968, Hirsch and Waugh added wired strain gauges to Harrington rods during spinal deformity correction and measured the axial load on the implant postoperatively.[5] However, percutaneous wires increased infection risk, tethered the patient to monitoring equipment, and made commercialization impractical.

Since then, there have been considerable advancements in wireless technology. Interbody fusion cages are potentially ideal devices for incorporating smart wireless monitoring technology. In 2007, Rohlmann and colleagues led the development of wirelessly powered spine implants with the first human trials.[6] Three vertebral body replacement cages using wireless power and telemetry monitoring were implanted into 3 patients, replacing fractured L1 vertebral bodies. Six load components were measured for several exercises in upright and lying positions within the first postoperative month (**Fig. 1**). The embedded sensors and inductive coils were hermetically sealed, protecting them from the surrounding biological fluids and tissue. High loads were found to act on the vertebral body replacement during

several exercises in the first month postoperatively. This guided their postoperative patient activities to reduce implant loads and the chance of implant subsidence.

The Persona IQ (Zimmer Biomet and Canary Medical) knee replacement system is an example of how wireless smart implants with sensors can bring benefits to patients. This system uses a smart implant located in the tibial stem that passively collects data on patient activity, knee range of motion, implant stability, and kinematic gait assessment.[7,8] Machine learning technology is used to compare each individual's functional recovery versus expectation and probe for gait abnormalities that can be mathematically correlated with specific complications of total knee arthroplasty.[7,8] Recent advancements in sensor and battery technologies have made it possible for Canary Medical to design a similar device small enough for inclusion in an interbody cage. The smart interbody spacer contains a 3-dimensional gyroscope, 3-dimensional accelerometer, step counter, Bluetooth transmission technology, and a pacemaker battery with enough power to collect daily, objective, functional data for 1 year and intermittent data for 20 years thereafter. There is nothing to wear or charge. Data are transmitted automatically every night from the implant to a base station in the patient's bedroom; relayed to a secure, closed-cloud system for further analysis; and displayed the following morning on the physician's and patient's computer or smart phone.[9]

Low-resolution readings (20 observations per second; ie, within the visual spectrum) collected from the gyroscope, accelerometer, and step counter are used to measure the patient's functional activity (step count, walking speed, distance, stride length, and cadence) continuously during waking hours (7 am to 10 pm). High-resolution readings (1600–3200 observations per second; ie, subvisual movement and vibration) are collected 3 times per day during active walking periods and used to calculate sagittal angle (posture), spinal range of motion, and implant fixation (loose implants vibrate during ambulation at a different frequency than implants firmly encased in bone). Data metrics are combined and analyzed by machine learning to estimate osteointegration and subsidence and to create predictive models for risk of infection, deep vein thrombosis, and hospital readmission. By extension, applying similar techniques to spinal implants could likewise bring benefits to the patient.

As exemplified in cardiac and neurostimulation devices and in the knee replacement system discussed previously, wireless battery-powered

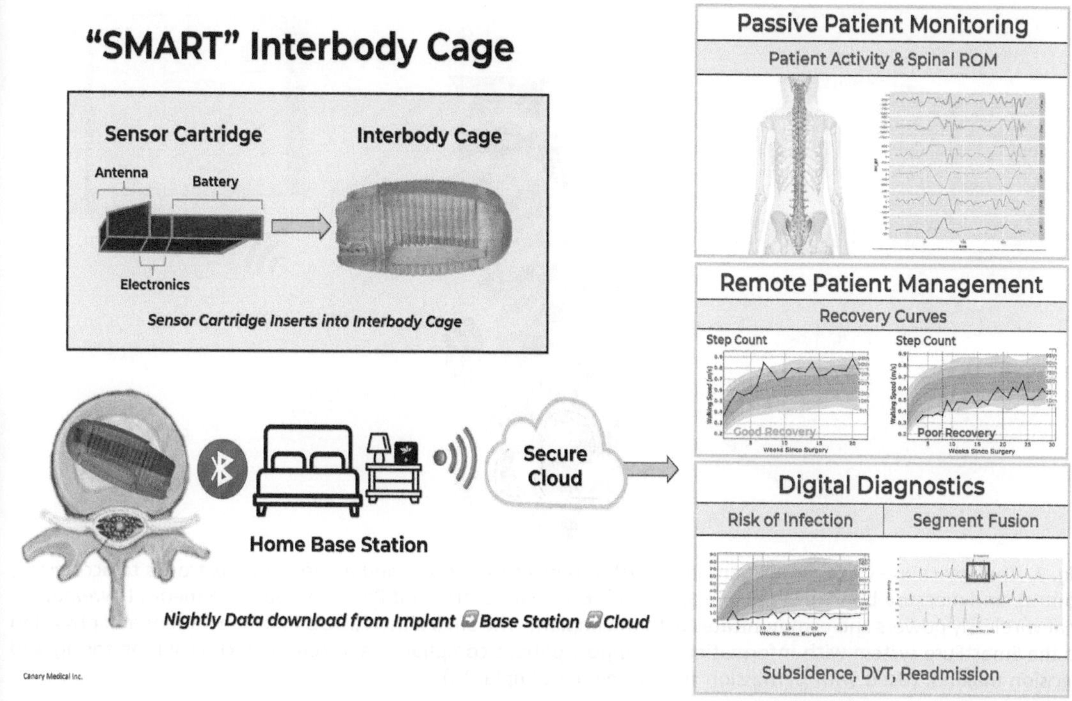

Fig. 1. Smart interbody cage, ecosystem, and data services and analytics (Canary Medical). Inset: A smart cartridge containing an antenna, sensors (3-dimensional gyroscope, 3-dimensional accelerometer, and step counter) and a power source (20-year pacemaker battery) inserts into a matching receptacle in the interbody cage without affecting structural integrity of the device. Ecosystem: Every night, data are transmitted using Bluetooth via an antenna sitting on the surface of the device (facing posteriorly), from the implant, through the tissue, and to a base station located in the patient's bedroom. Raw data are sent by Wi-Fi to a secure, closed cloud for further analysis and transmission to the doctor and patient the following morning. Data Services and Analytics: Activity metrics (step count, walking speed, distance, stride length, and cadence) provide insight into levels of patient activity and recovery. Range of motion (ROM), posture, and implant movement and vibration are calculated as indicators of spinal function and segment fixation. Recovery curves compare observed patient progress to expected population (matched by sex and age) values. Machine learning is applied to the collected data to predict the relative risk of developing complications such as nonunion, subsidence, infection, hospital readmission, and deep vein thrombosis (DVT). (Used with permission from Canary Medical.)

sensor and telemetry technology has been on the market for years. Unfortunately, battery-powered systems have limitations for spinal implant use.[10] Spinal intervertebral spacers and screws are too small to be able to house large batteries, and small batteries have a short life. Cardiac and neurostimulation pulse generators use subcutaneous batteries that are replaceable with simple outpatient surgery or recharged with subcutaneous wireless transmission coils. Orthopedic implants, and spine implants in particular, are much deeper in the body or buried in bone. Because of this, orthopedic device batteries cannot be easily replaced or charged using common wireless power transmission techniques. In addition, batteries are at risk of failing and leaking of oxidative chemicals, which must be considered, because orthopedic implants are subjected to significant mechanical loading.

Therefore, smart spinal implants will benefit from a power supply that requires no implanted batteries. In medical devices, this is often achieved using inductive coupling. Inductive coupling powers the implant with an external coil that is attached to or worn on the body. This external electrical coil is coupled by means of an electromagnetic field to a coil embedded in the implant. This coupling enables wireless power transfer to the internal coil and ultimately to the implant.

One of the challenges with wireless smart spine implants is that the spinal vertebrae are located deep in the body, up to 14 cm from the skin in some patients. The implants themselves are often small, giving little room for electronics and antenna within the implants. Wireless power transmission efficiency is affected by transmission distance and antenna size. Because wireless spinal implants require long distances and small antennae,

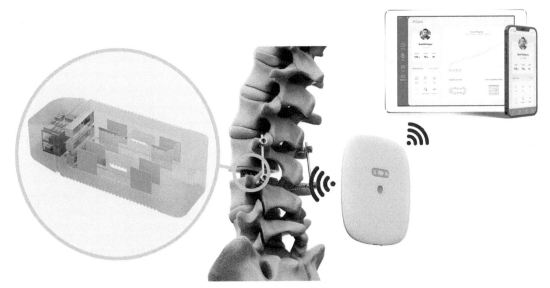

Fig. 2. The SmartFuse CAGE (Intelligent Implants) uses electrical signals and an array of electrodes to accelerate, control, and measure bone growth. The SmartFuse External Control and Power module is a medical "wearable" that wirelessly powers and communicates with the implant. The SmartFuse CLOUD links the patient and physician to the SmartFuse system with information to support patient compliance and real-time clinical monitoring and decision making. (Used with permission from Intelligent Implants.)

the amount of energy that can be practically transmitted is small.

Thus, electronics developed for spine implants need to be very low power, miniaturized, and packaged to fit safely within small spine implants that can withstand the substantial loads transmitted through the spine. In addition, the smart implants must be compatible with newer techniques used in minimally invasive surgery.

A wireless inductive-coupled and cloud-connected electrotherapeutic technology that uses electrical signals to accelerate, control, and remotely monitor bone growth is currently being developed (SmartFuse; Intelligent Implants) (**Fig. 2**).[11] Using an array of electrodes to precisely stimulate and measure bone directly at the desired site of healing, this technology causes the body to "3D print" bone in situ exactly where it is needed. An array of electrodes on the surface of the implant enables spatial control of bone growth. It equally improves diagnostic capabilities by being able to make higher-fidelity measurements of bone growth and provide much more information to the surgeon regarding bone growth within and around the implant.

An alternative method to power smart implants that could avoid the challenges of wireless power transmission is energy harvesting. Energy harvesting involves converting kinetic energy of gross movements, such as walking, to electrical energy, effectively creating a self-powered system.

Implants are being developed that create small pulses of current with each step that patients take to stimulate bone growth in the spine at the site of implantation.[12] These implants are designed to use dynamic compression forces transmitted through the implant as the patient ambulates and transform that force into energy pulses.

Smart spine implants could improve implant insertion. Current insertion techniques are guided by tactile feedback, imaging, and assistance from robots. Sensors and impedance measurements may provide real-time feedback during spinal surgeries, helping surgeons achieve more accurate site preparation, placement, and alignment of spinal implants. A smart spinal implant could provide a surgical robot with additional feedback to improve surgical outcomes. Impedance measurements collected by the implant could provide feedback on endplate preparation, the quality of bone, and other factors. Currently, there are no preclinical or clinical smart implants with this ability.

In addition to power and packaging challenges, obstacles to widespread use of smart spine implants include the limited accuracy of sensors, the difficulty in obtaining useful data, the increased cost of implants, and privacy concerns.

All current clinical sensor designs measure mechanical loading, the environment immediately surrounding the implant, or the motion of the implant as it performs in vivo. One can infer the loads exerted on the vertebral body and the posterior elements, but these inferences may not accurately correspond to the forces and moments acting on the spine. Likewise, the immediate environment or motion of the implant must be correlated with the state of the spine as a whole and the patient's health and recovery. Output from sensors in smart spinal implants will need to be translated into useful, actionable data for the surgeon and health care providers.

Surgeons must not be overloaded with these data. This is a challenge and opportunity for the medical device industry to create solutions that highlight useful data and create efficient, actionable workflows. The ability to remotely monitor patients has a huge potential to increase the efficiency of health care resources. A major flaw in current treatment regimens is the lack of long-term postsurgical follow-up. Current technology does not allow for long-term patient observation because of cost, resource availability, and the desire to limit patient's exposure to radiation from excessive imaging. By enabling automated remote collection of data, smart implant technology can remove these obstacles and enable long-term, personalized patient follow-up.

Smart spinal implants will initially be more expensive than standard implants. Justifying this higher initial cost will require a cost-benefit analysis with a demonstrated net reduction in health care costs. Reduction of costs by decreasing postoperative complications must be demonstrated with data. The advantages of automated long-term patient monitoring must likewise be demonstrated.

The regulatory path for smart implants also represents a challenge. The US Food and Drug Administration (FDA) is generally supportive of smart spine implants including remote monitoring of patients. The FDA breakthrough device pathway is also available to streamline regulatory approval of this type of cutting-edge technology.[13] Even with this support, the regulatory path to human use and commercial release is lengthy and costly.

Connected spine implants also bring security hazards that, in theory, could put patients at risk. Data from the implants could bring the risk of loss of privacy. Furthermore, difficult questions, including access to this information, how long it is kept, and the extent to which the patient is informed regarding the implant status, must be answered.[14]

SUMMARY

Smart spine implants have the potential to revolutionize the field of spinal health care by offering personalized, data-driven treatments, continuous monitoring, active influence on the healing process, and improved patient outcomes. However, it is important to note that although these technologies show promise, availability and widespread adoption represent considerable technical and regulatory approval challenges.

FINANCIAL SUPPORT

None.

ACKNOWLEDGMENTS

The authors thank the staff of Neuroscience Publications at Barrow Neurological Institute for assistance with manuscript preparation.

DISCLOSURE

Dr R.K.J. Murphy holds equity in Intelligent Implants, Therapha, Consultant Stryker, Nuvasive, Icotec, and Zimvie Spine.

REFERENCES

1. Ledet EH, Liddle B, Kradinova K, et al. Smart implants in orthopedic surgery, improving patient outcomes: a review. Innov Entrep Health 2018;5:41–51.
2. Kim SJ, Wang T, Pelletier MH, et al. 'SMART' implantable devices for spinal implants: a systematic review on current and future trends. J Spine Surg 2022; 8(1):117–31.
3. Iyengar KP, Kariya AD, Botchu R, et al. Significant capabilities of SMART sensor technology and their applications for Industry 4.0 in trauma and orthopaedics. Sensors International 2022;3:100163.
4. Ernst M, Baumgartner H, Dobele S, et al. Clinical feasibility of fracture healing assessment through continuous monitoring of implant load. J Biomech 2021;116:110188.
5. Hirsch C, Waugh T. The introduction of force measurements guiding instrumental correction of scoliosis. Acta Orthop Scand 1968;39(2):136–44.
6. Rohlmann A, Gabel U, Graichen F, et al. An instrumented implant for vertebral body replacement that measures loads in the anterior spinal column. Med Eng Phys 2007;29(5):580–5.
7. Becker's Spine Review. What could smart implants look like in spine? Available at: https://www. beckersspine.com/spine/57134-what-could-smart-implants-look-like-in-spine.html. Accessed June 15, 2023.
8. Carroll K, Gemmell K, Aubin P. The sensor enabled TKA: a novel approach to gait analysis (abstract 7657). 2022.
9. Cushner FD, Sculco PK, Long WJ. The talking knee is a reality: what your knee can tell you after total

knee arthroplasty. J Orthopaedic Experience & Innovation 2022. https://doi.org/10.60118/001c.35270.

10. Lowe M, Nguyen L, Patel DJ. A review of the recent advances of cardiac pacemaker technology in handling complications. J Long Term Eff Med Implants 2023;33(4):21–9.

11. Murphy R, John K, Zellmer ER, et al. System and method to alter bone growth in a targeted spatial region for the use with implants. Patent Application 2023;211, 18/097.

12. Friis EA, Krech E, Cadel E, et al. Inventors; stacked piezoelectric energy harvester. Patent Application 2021;262, 17/045.

13. Baumann AP, O'Neill C, Owens MC, et al. FDA public workshop: orthopaedic sensing, measuring, and advanced reporting technology (SMART) devices. J Orthop Res 2021;39(1):22–9.

14. Pycroft L, Aziz TZ. Security of implantable medical devices with wireless connections: the dangers of cyber-attacks. Expert Rev Med Devices 2018; 15(6):403–6.

Digital Phenotyping, Wearables, and Outcomes

Anshul Ratnaparkhi, BS[a], Joel Beckett, MD, MHS[a,b],*

KEYWORDS

- Wearables • Digital phenotyping • Spine surgery • Artificial intelligence • Machine learning

KEY POINTS

- Digital phenotyping facilitates constant and unobtrusive patient monitoring, providing holistic information relevant to spine surgery.
- Artificial intelligence and machine learning can integrate data from multiple sources— including imaging, patient history, spatiotemporal data, and other relevant biomarkers— to identify associations not currently known in medical practice.
- Wearable devices and digital phenotyping will provide objective data for clinical decision-making.
- To deploy remote patient monitoring in routine clinical practice, the technologies introduced must be seamlessly integrated into the current clinical workflow.

INTRODUCTION

In 1965, Gordon Moore proclaimed that the number of transistors in an integrated circuit would double every two years.[1,2] This observation, known as Moore's Law, would hold for the next four decades. The rapid growth in computational ability has paved the way for the digitization of contemporary society. Today, more than 85% of Americans own a smartphone, compared with just 35% in 2011.[3] The explosion of smartphone ownership has been coupled with immense global technological innovation, putting highly accurate accelerometers, global positioning system (GPS) tracking, and even light detection and ranging sensors[4,5] into our pockets. This opens the door for measuring various biomarkers, including spatiotemporal variables, heart rate, and skin conductance, ultimately facilitating remote patient monitoring on an unprecedented level. This wealth of relevant diagnostic information may help physicians, scientists, and patients revolutionize health care.

Monitoring the human-technology interaction is at the crux of the digital phenotype. This concept builds on the extended phenotype, the notion that

phenotypes should not be confined to only biological processes.[6] Coined by Richard Dawkins, the extended phenotype suggests that an organism's direct or indirect effects on its environment and other organisms should be included in its phenotype.[7] This premise is expanded to include our interaction with technology via the digital phenotype, defined as the "moment-by-moment quantification of the individual-level human phenotype in situ using data from personal digital devices."[8] Digital phenotyping will provide continuous and instantaneous insight into patient well-being in the real world by harnessing the power of smartphones and other wearable devices. This allows for the unobtrusive capture of objective and longitudinal metrics on physical activity, mobility, cognition, communication, and other core aspects of human health.

DISCUSSION
Overview of Existing Wearable Technology

Typically, patients present to their primary care provider after the onset of symptoms that affect their quality of life. The treating physician is then

[a] Department of Neurosurgery, David Geffen School of Medicine, University of California Los Angeles; [b] David Geffen School of Medicine, University of California Los Angeles
* Corresponding author. Department of Neurosurgery, David Geffen School of Medicine, University of California Los Angeles, 300 Stein Plaza, Ste 535, Los Angeles, CA 90095.
E-mail address: JBeckett@mednet.ucla.edu

Neurosurg Clin N Am 35 (2024) 235–241
https://doi.org/10.1016/j.nec.2023.11.009
1042-3680/24/© 2023 Elsevier Inc. All rights reserved.

charged with making a diagnosis by combining clinical presentation, imaging, patient history, and other diagnostic tests. Once a decision is reached, the patient follows up with their clinician at intervals, creating snapshots of their health profile at each consultation. For instance, the gold standard for evaluating functional recovery can be quantified as clinically reported or subjective patient-reported outcomes, such as the visual analog scale and Oswestry Disability Index.[9,10] Thus, robust and objective functional outcome assessments in spine surgery are needed.

Wearable versions of laboratory-based technologies have immense potential to provide valuable diagnostic and prognostic information from daily ambulatory monitoring. Medical devices have demonstrated success in disease monitoring, from biosensors for diabetes management[11,12] to wearable Zio patch systems[13] and smartwatch electrocardiograms (ECGs)[14] for remote cardiac monitoring. Both implantable and wearable sensors are used more frequently as spine surgery transitions into a data-driven field. Strain gauges have long been used to monitor lumbar strain in cadavers[15] and animal models.[16] These sensors have recently demonstrated in vitro success.[17] La Barbera and colleagues measured the loading distribution following pedicle subtraction osteotomies and the strain caused by posterior fixation and anterior interbody fusion.[18]

Perhaps the sensors most relevant to spine surgery are inertial measurement units (IMUs). These devices combine accelerometers and gyroscopes to measure acceleration and angular velocity.[19] IMUs are highly relevant devices for gait analysis, a critical component of the neurologic examination that provides a wealth of diagnostic information helpful in identifying and monitoring disease progression.[20] These sensors are accurate and validated against the gold standard for motion capture—marker-based optoelectrical tracking.[21] Marker-based tracking is inherently inconvenient for capturing motion in routine clinical practice and at-home rehabilitation settings due to the need to decorate subjects with reflective markers and record them under controlled lighting.[22,23] The ease of operation and low-profile nature of IMUs provide the flexibility to wear in real-world conditions. This opens the door for managing patient activities of daily living, providing continuous data collection, and monitoring in sports and other movement-intensive domains.[24]

Modern smartphones have built-in accelerometers, gyroscopes, and GPS tracking, allowing for relevant physiologic data to be captured.[25] The consumer-grade wearable technology industry has also seen recent economic growth and technological innovation. Smartwatch capabilities have expanded from measuring individuals' step count and heart rate to more complicated tasks, ranging from detecting atrial fibrillation via abnormal pulse detection[26,27] to predicting purchase intent using the built-in electrocardiogram (EKG) feature on Apple Watches.[28] The contemporary smartwatch monitors complex variables implicated in disease diagnosis and prognosis, such as gait, body temperature, sleep–wake cycles, heart rate, and overall activity level.[29] Combining a patient's physical activity, spatiotemporal measurements, and vitals measured by smartphones and smartwatches with existing clinical data can form a comprehensive package of patient health.

Objective Biomarkers for Spine Surgery

The decision-making process in neurosurgery often dwells in shades of gray rather than stark black-and-white choices such as whether or not to operate. Instead, decision making involves strategic deliberations regarding the timing and method of surgical intervention, for example, the management of degenerative lumbar conditions, in which surgeons can access a wide array of treatment modalities. Present protocols span from endoscopic to traditional decompression procedures to various fusion techniques. These include the posterior lumbar interbody fusion, the transforaminal lumbar interbody fusion, the anterior lumbar interbody fusion, and the lateral lumbar interbody fusion. Although each technique has idiosyncratic pearls and pitfalls, most surgeons tend to perform the operation they were trained in, irrespective of pathology or operative levels.[30] This is, in part, a result of the paucity of in vivo[31] and class 1 and 2 biomechanical data comparing surgical techniques.[30] As spine surgery grows and new surgical procedures are developed, objective metrics to measure and compare patient outcomes are increasingly needed.

One domain for wearable devices and digital phenotyping is monitoring cervical spondylotic myelopathy (CSM). CSM is a progressive disease defined by degenerative changes to the intervertebral disks, facets, vertebrae, and associated ligaments[32] that engenders myelopathy via compression of neural and vascular elements. The progression of CSM correlates with deteriorating clinical presentation, such as gait instability and fine motor control difficulty. The degree of stenosis that requires decompression needs to be better defined, and it is currently debated whether surgery is the right course of treatment for patients presenting with CSM.[33] Disease prognosis via wearables offers an opportunity for monitoring the progression of this disease. Gait analysis has already demonstrated success in tracking the progression of other conditions, including Parkinson's disease,[34] and may facilitate more appropriate CSM treatment. Integrating wearables to monitor CSM and other surgical pathology may increase the percentage of patients that benefit from surgical intervention.

Remote Patient Monitoring

Spine surgery represents the third largest expenditure in national health care, reflecting its significance and impact.[35] The associated risks and outcomes of these operations, however, warrant attention. Specifically, there is a substantial complication rate of 26% across all types of spine surgery[36] and an early readmission rate of 9.4% for elective procedures.[37] These complications could lead to serious health consequences if overlooked or improperly managed. Hence, it is paramount to maximize surgical outcomes through meticulous surgical procedures and rigorous postoperative monitoring and rehabilitation.[38] These postsurgery steps are crucial in the patient's recovery journey, emphasizing that the surgery itself is just one component of a successful treatment process.

It has long been known that ambulation trends and activity levels are important biomarkers of a patient's functional recovery following surgery: numerous studies have demonstrated that increased postoperative ambulation is correlated with improved patient outcomes, including decreased length of stay, discharge disposition, and chances of readmission.[39,40] Despite this, there is a lack of accurate and objective mobility data used for postoperative management.[41] Instead, physicians rely on subjective metrics for ambulatory and overall fitness status, such as patient-reported outcomes and the ODI scores.[42] Data-driven, clinically relevant measurements are needed to quantify patient fitness and mobile status. Wearable devices and digital phenotyping have the potential to capture this data, providing a better insight into patient recovery following surgery. This has been exemplified in numerous studies: the Fitbit device has demonstrated that it can track adult spinal deformity (ASD) patients throughout their care. In this study, Haglin and colleagues demonstrated that the changes in a patient's activity level could be monitored using the step count feature of a smartwatch.[43] As tracked by wearables, increased activity has also been demonstrated in a physiotherapy setting in a cohort of 26 patients diagnosed with nonspecific low back pain (LBP)[44] and other specialties.[45] Significantly, the trends in the recorded movement were correlated with overall clinical status and radiographic severity, highlighting the validity of using wearables for functional evaluation.

Remote patient monitoring using wearables can also evaluate patient recovery directly. Spinal fusions are some of the most common surgeries performed and are only increasing in prevalence,[46] yet operations are plagued with high complication, failure, and revision rates. One of the most frequent causes of revision, specifically in patients with ASD, is incomplete fusion.[47] Although radiographic fusion grade has not impacted the health-related quality of life in ASD patients,[48] implantable sensors can augment postoperative patient evaluation via traditional radiographic evaluation.[49] These sensors have successfully provided real-time postoperative recovery data.[16,50] Rod strain and fracture, caused by an excessive force being placed on the spine,[51] is relatively common morbidity in spine surgery. Rod failure occurred in 9% of ASD patients and 22% of pedicle subtraction osteotomy patients within 1 year.[52] Thus, there is a need to monitor rod strain in patients and better understand how load-bearing changes in patients undergoing various operations to limit this adverse outcome. Deriving additional methods for evaluating fusion progress may benefit spine surgeons and patients.

Personalized Medicine

Ecologically valid measurements on a patient-specific level may provide the most accurate and beneficial way to understand the association between clinical presentation and disease management. For instance, many cases of LBP are related to or aggravated by activities of daily living.[53] By integrating the tracking of movements related to flare-ups of LBP with other risk factors detectable by wearable devices, such as physical activity and sleep patterns, we could devise a more personalized approach to managing LBP. This tailored strategy has the potential to significantly reduce the frequency and intensity of LBP for each patient. This implies that merging wearable technology with medical intervention may revolutionize how we alleviate chronic conditions such as LBP, leading to more effective and patient-specific solutions.

A data-driven approach to personalized health care delivers the metrics required for patients to play a more significant role in clinical decision-making. Shared decision-making (SDM) revolves around constructing a physician–patient relationship to understand the patient's values, preferences, and needs while serving as an educator on the risks, benefits, and alternative options.[54] It has become a cornerstone of modern medical practice and is recognized as essential to patient-focused care.[55] Recent studies on remote patient monitoring have demonstrated that patients benefit when consultations revolve around personalized data.[56,57] As spine surgery advances, understanding the patient's treatment goals becomes increasingly essential when deciding not just on invasive or conservative treatment, but also on the technique and timing of the operation. The data collected via wearable devices and digital phenotyping provide the data-driven foundation for patients to participate optimally in SDM.

A Better Understanding of Disease

Synthesizing patient data across multiple data streams is now possible due to the raw power of modern-day computing that facilitates the observation and weighing of a limitless amount of data.[58] Artificial intelligence (AI) has significant potential to integrate multiple data sources, including patient imaging, electronic medical records, and objective data captured using wearables.[59]

Machine learning holds immense potential to unify multiple data streams, effectively characterizing the factors influencing disease progression from an asymptomatic stage to a pathologic phenotype.[59] By systematically analyzing these diverse data sources, machine learning algorithms can discern intricate patterns and correlations that may be imperceptible to the human eye. This can provide valuable insights into the transition of diseases from subclinical to severe stages, which can guide more precise, timely, and personalized therapeutic interventions. One such opportunity is predicting, detecting, and monitoring proximal junction kyphosis (PJK). PJK is a constant concern for surgeons performing spinal deformity surgery as it can rapidly progress to proximal junction failure (PJF), requiring revision surgery. The pathogenesis of PJK and the mechanisms that cause PJK to develop into PJF are largely unknown and multifactorial. As a result, the current classifications of PJK and PJF are incomplete and have unique deficits.[60–62] Combining patient phenotyping mechanisms, such as intraoperative rod monitoring, postural positioning tracking, and activity levels, with existing methods, including dual-energy x-ray absorptiometry, imaging reports, and clinical presentation, may lead to a comprehensive risk assessment for PJK and PJF. This holistic understanding may assist physicians in treating their patients better and mitigate the burden on the health care system.

Limitations

The integration of wearable device data and digital phenotyping holds significant promise for advancing precision and personalized medicine; however, numerous steps must be taken before these technologies can be implemented on a widespread basis.

A crucial aspect to consider is that the patient is the primary gatekeeper of data collection. The efficacy of wearable devices and digital phenotyping depends on the patient's willingness to use these devices consistently and their comfort with data sharing. Despite studies revealing relatively low attrition rates with wearable technologies compared with other methods, potential concerns about sharing personal data with medical professionals and third-party entities can pose significant obstacles to the broad application of digital phenotyping in medicine.[63,64] Factors such as inadequate privacy disclosures have been flagged as areas of concern regarding data sharing.[65] This challenge is further complicated as manufacturers of smart devices often need more support in sharing raw metrics. These hurdles indicate the traditionally slow pace of integrating emerging technologies into clinical practice.[64] We must thoughtfully navigate these issues to ensure the clinical significance of wearables and digital phenotyping. The formalization and ethical use of technology need to be comprehensively considered and appropriately addressed to realize the full potential of these digital tools in health care.

Data generated via wearables are typically created by nonprofessionals in nonstandard ways. Data accuracy and consistency are worth disucssing as measurement systems in smartphones and wearable devices are less precise than laboratory-grade equipment captured under standardized conditions. This creates the potential for errors via unequal sampling, data absence, or anomalous data unrelated to an individual's behavior. There is also a higher chance of human and technological error leading to inaccuracy.[66] No current strategy exists for addressing these issues,[66] and nonstandard, ambiguous data should not be the sole determinant of medical decisions. Instead, we believe that accruing data in nonstandard ways outside of clinical practice has a unique value that complements more traditional data collection. Remote patient monitoring better reflects the patient's status in the real world and thus provides additional data for physicians to consider when deciding treatment outcomes. These metrics can fill information gaps for health management, create new workflows for remote care, and develop clinical decisions in real time.[59] Ultimately, we believe that patient-generated health data via wearables and digital phenotyping should augment clinical practice to create a more holistic representation of patient health.

SUMMARY

The advent of wearable devices and digital phenotyping has unlocked the potential for a genuinely data-centric approach to spine surgery. The varied and rapidly growing range of wearables—encompassing everything from smartphones to portable laboratory-grade equipment—generates a wealth of ecologically valid data points relevant to spine surgery. Leveraging recent advancements in artificial intelligence and machine learning, the enormous volume of data collected via these devices can be meticulously analyzed and effectively used for clinical decision-making. This data-driven approach does not merely empower physicians to quantify disease more accurately: it also enables the integration of novel data streams, such as activity monitoring and gait analysis, into traditional clinical practice. The result is a more comprehensive understanding of patient health and disease status, as it harmoniously combines conventional clinical wisdom with cutting-edge technology and big data analytics. Hence, the future of spine surgery—and indeed medicine—could be characterized by this seamless blend of old and new, thereby fostering personalized, precise, and holistic health care solutions.

CLINICS CARE POINTS

- Combining the increased amount of objective data generated via wearables and advancements in artificial intelligence can create digital phenotypes of patients, disease states, and treatments.

- Machine learning has the potential to augment existing medical practice by uncovering new associations between clinical presentation, patient history, imaging, pathology reports, and other diagnostic tests.

- The utility of these additional data is to provide a more holistic understanding of patient and disease states, augmenting—not replacing—existing clinical workflows.

DISCLOSURES

The authors have no relevant disclosures to the present work.

REFERENCES

1. Moore GE. No exponential is forever: but "Forever" can be delayed! (semiconductor industry). In: 2003 IEEE International Solid-State Circuits Conference, 2003. Digest of Technical Papers. ISSCC. IEEE; 2003. 10.1109/issue.2003.1234194.
2. Moore G. Cramming more components onto integrated circuits (1965). In: Ideas that created the future. The MIT Press; 2021. p. 261–6.
3. Mobile Fact Sheet. Pew Research Center: Internet, Science & Tech. Published April 7, 2021. Accessed April 27, 2023. https://www.pewresearch.org/internet/fact-sheet/mobile/.
4. Mikalai Z, Andrey D, Hawas HS, et al. Human body measurement with the iPhone 12 Pro LiDAR scanner. In: International conference on textile and apparel innovation (ICTAI 2021). AIP Publishing; 2022. https://doi.org/10.1063/5.0078310.
5. Bhandarkar AR, Bhandarkar S, Jarrah RM, et al. Smartphone-based light detection and ranging for remote patient evaluation and monitoring. Cureus 2021;13(8):e16886.
6. Dawkins R. The extended phenotype: the gene as the unit of selection. Oxford, Oxfordshire: Freeman; 1982.
7. Hunter P. The revival of the extended phenotype. EMBO Rep 2018;19(7):e46477.
8. Onnela JP, Rauch SL. Harnessing Smartphone-Based Digital Phenotyping to Enhance Behavioral and Mental Health. Neuropsychopharmacology 2016;41(7):1691–6.
9. Boaro A, Leung J, Reeder HT, et al. Smartphone GPS signatures of patients undergoing spine surgery correlate with mobility and current gold standard outcome measures. J Neurosurg Spine 2021; 35(6):796–806.
10. Panda N, Perez N, Tsangaris E, et al. Enhancing Patient-Centered Surgical Care With Mobile Health Technology. J Surg Res 2022;274:178–84.
11. Lee H, Choi TK, Lee YB, et al. A graphene-based electrochemical device with thermoresponsive microneedles for diabetes monitoring and therapy. Nat Nanotechnol 2016;11(6):566–72.
12. Lipani L, Dupont BGR, Doungmene F, et al. Non-invasive, transdermal, path-selective and specific glucose monitoring via a graphene-based platform. Nat Nanotechnol 2018;13(6):504–11.
13. Yenikomshian M, Jarvis J, Patton C, et al. Cardiac arrhythmia detection outcomes among patients monitored with the Zio patch system: a systematic literature review. Curr Med Res Opin 2019;35(10): 1659–70.
14. Isakadze N, Martin SS. How useful is the smartwatch ECG? Trends Cardiovasc Med 2020;30(7): 442–8.
15. Szivek JA, Roberto RF, Slack JM, et al. An implantable strain measurement system designed to detect spine fusion. Preliminary results from a biomechanical and in vivo study. Spine 2002;27:487–97.
16. Windolf M, Heumann M, Varjas V, et al. Continuous rod load monitoring to assess spinal fusion status-

pilot in vivo data in sheep. Medicina (Kaunas). 2022; 58(7):899.

17. Szivek JA, Roberto RF, Margolis DS. In vivo strain measurements from hardware and lamina during spine fusion. J Biomed Mater Res B Appl Biomater 2005;75(2):243–50.

18. La Barbera L, Wilke HJ, Ruspi ML, et al. Load-sharing biomechanics of lumbar fixation and fusion with pedicle subtraction osteotomy. Sci Rep 2021; 11(1):3595.

19. Fong DTP, Chan YY. The use of wearable inertial motion sensors in human lower limb biomechanics studies: a systematic review. Sensors 2010;10(12): 11556–65.

20. Klöpfer-Krämer I, Brand A, Wackerle H, et al. Gait analysis - Available platforms for outcome assessment. Injury 2020;51(Suppl 2):S90–6.

21. Bailey CA, Uchida TK, Nantel J, et al. Validity and Sensitivity of an Inertial Measurement Unit-Driven Biomechanical Model of Motor Variability for Gait. Sensors 2021;(22):21. https://doi.org/10.3390/s21227690.

22. Alfakir A, Arrowsmith C, Burns D, et al. Detection of low back physiotherapy exercises with inertial sensors and machine learning: Algorithm development and validation. JMIR Rehabil Assist Technol 2022; 9(3):e38689.

23. Sigal L, Balan AO, Black MJ. HumanEva: Synchronized Video and Motion Capture Dataset and Baseline Algorithm for Evaluation of Articulated Human Motion. Int J Comput Vis 2010;87(1–2):4–27.

24. Hafer JF, Mihy JA, Hunt A, et al. Lower Extremity Inverse Kinematics Results Differ Between Inertial Measurement Unit- and Marker-Derived Gait Data. J Appl Biomech 2023;1–10.

25. Straczkiewicz M, James P, Onnela JP. A systematic review of smartphone-based human activity recognition methods for health research. npj Digital Medicine 2021;4(1). https://doi.org/10.1038/s41746-021-00514-4.

26. Tajrishi FZ, Chitsazan M, Chitsazan M, et al. Smartwatch for the detection of atrial fibrillation. Crit Pathw Cardiol 2019;18(4):176–84.

27. Wyatt KD, Poole LR, Mullan AF, et al. Clinical evaluation and diagnostic yield following evaluation of abnormal pulse detected using Apple Watch. J Am Med Inf Assoc 2020;27(9):1359–63.

28. Chang RI, Tsai CY, Chung P. Smartwatch sensors with deep learning to predict the purchase intentions of online shoppers. Sensors 2022;23(1):430.

29. Costa N, Smits EJ, Kasza J, et al. Are objective measures of sleep and sedentary behaviours related to low back pain flares? Pain 2022;163(9):1829–37.

30. Mobbs RJ, Phan K, Malham G, et al. Lumbar interbody fusion: techniques, indications and comparison of interbody fusion options including PLIF, TLIF, MI-TLIF, OLIF/ATP, LLIF and ALIF. J Spine Surg 2015;1(1):2–18.

31. Ramakrishna VAS, Chamoli U, Rajan G, et al. Smart orthopaedic implants: A targeted approach for continuous postoperative evaluation in the spine. J Biomech 2020;104(109690):109690.

32. McCormick JR, Sama AJ, Schiller NC, et al. Cervical spondylotic myelopathy: A guide to diagnosis and management. J Am Board Fam Med 2020;33(2): 303–13.

33. Ghogawala Z, Benzel EC, Riew KD, et al. Surgery vs conservative care for cervical spondylotic myelopathy: Surgery is appropriate for progressive myelopathy. Neurosurgery 2015;62(Supplement 1):56–61.

34. Biase L di, di Biase L, Di Santo A, et al. Gait Analysis in Parkinson's Disease: An Overview of the Most Accurate Markers for Diagnosis and Symptoms Monitoring. Sensors 2020;20(12):3529.

35. Dieleman JL, Baral R, Birger M, et al. US spending on personal health care and public health, 1996-2013. JAMA 2016;316(24):2627.

36. Lange N, Stadtmüller T, Scheibel S, et al. Analysis of risk factors for perioperative complications in spine surgery. Sci Rep 2022;12(1):14350.

37. Adogwa O, Elsamadicy AA, Han JL, et al. 30-day readmission after spine surgery: An analysis of 1400 consecutive spine surgery patients. Spine (Phila Pa 1976) 2016. https://doi.org/10.1097/BRS.0000000000001779.

38. Morimoto T, Hirata H, Ueno M, et al. Digital Transformation Will Change Medical Education and Rehabilitation in Spine Surgery. Medicina 2022;58(4). https://doi.org/10.3390/medicina58040508.

39. Outline Images Download Cite Share Favorites Permissions RESEARCH-HUMAN-CLINICAL STUDIES: SPINE Validation of the Benefits of Ambulation Within 8 Hours of Elective Cervical and Lumbar Surgery: A Michigan Spine Surgery Improvement Collaborative Study.

40. Zakaria HM, Bazydlo M, Schultz L, et al. Ambulation on postoperative day #0 is associated with decreased morbidity and adverse events after elective lumbar spine surgery: Analysis from the Michigan Spine Surgery Improvement Collaborative (MSSIC). Neurosurgery 2020;87(2):320–8.

41. Stienen MN, Rezaii PG, Ho AL, et al. Objective activity tracking in spine surgery: a prospective feasibility study with a low-cost consumer grade wearable accelerometer. Sci Rep 2020;10(1):4939.

42. Krummel TM. The Rise of Wearable Technology in Health Care. JAMA Netw Open 2019;2(2): e187672.

43. Haglin JM, Godzik J, Mauria R, et al. Continuous Activity Tracking Using a Wrist-Mounted Device in Adult Spinal Deformity: A Proof of Concept Study. World Neurosurg 2019;122:349–54.

44. Alzahrani H, Mackey M, Stamatakis E, et al. Wearables-based walking program in addition to usual physiotherapy care for the management of patients

with low back pain at medium or high risk of chronicity: A pilot randomized controlled trial. PLoS One 2021;16(8):e0256459.

45. Pandrangi VC, Jorizzo M, Shah S, et al. Monitoring postoperative ambulation and sleep after head and neck surgery: Feasibility and utility study using wearable devices. Head Neck 2022;44(12): 2744–52.

46. Al Jammal OM, Delavar A, Maguire KR, et al. National trends in the surgical management of lumbar spinal stenosis in adult spinal deformity patients. Spine (Phila Pa 1976) 2019;44(23):E1369–78.

47. Cho W, Mason JR, Smith JS, et al. Failure of lumbopelvic fixation after long construct fusions in patients with adult spinal deformity: clinical and radiographic risk factors. J Neurosurg Spine 2013;19(4):445–53.

48. Ailon T, Hamilton DK, Klineberg E, et al. Radiographic fusion grade does not impact health-related quality of life in the absence of instrumentation failure for patients undergoing posterior instrumented fusion for adult spinal deformity. World Neurosurg 2018;117:e1–7.

49. Barri K, Zhang Q, Mehta D, et al. Studying the Feasibility of Postoperative Monitoring of Spinal Fusion Progress Using a Self-Powered Fowler-Nordheim Sensor-Data-Logger. IEEE Trans Biomed Eng 2022; 69(2):710–7.

50. Aebersold JW, Hnat WP, Voor MJ, et al. Development of a strain transferring sensor housing for a lumbar spinal fusion detection system. J Med Device 2007;1(2):159–64.

51. Mushlin HM, Shea P, Brooks DM, et al. The effect of sacroiliac fusion and pelvic fixation on rod strain in thoracolumbar fusion constructs: A biomechanical investigation. Spine (Phila Pa 1976) 2021;46(14): E769–75.

52. Smith JS, Shaffrey E, Klineberg E, et al. Prospective multicenter assessment of risk factors for rod fracture following surgery for adult spinal deformity. J Neurosurg Spine 2014;21(6):994–1003.

53. Papi E, Koh WS, McGregor AH. Wearable technology for spine movement assessment: A systematic review. J Biomech 2017;64:186–97.

54. Rabi DM, Kunneman M, Montori VM. When guidelines recommend shared decision-making. JAMA 2020;323(14):1345–6.

55. Forner D, Noel CW, Shuman AG, et al. Shared decision-making in head and neck surgery: A review. JAMA Otolaryngol Head Neck Surg 2020; 146(9):839–44.

56. Austin L, Sharp CA, van der Veer SN, et al. Providing "the bigger picture": benefits and feasibility of integrating remote monitoring from smartphones into the electronic health record. Rheumatology (Oxford) 2020;59(2):367–78.

57. Prasse T, Yap N, Sivakanthan S, et al. Remote patient monitoring following full endoscopic spine surgery: feasibility and patient satisfaction. J Neurosurg Spine 2023;1–10.

58. Buch VH, Ahmed I, Maruthappu M. Artificial intelligence in medicine: current trends and future possibilities. Br J Gen Pract 2018;68(668):143–4.

59. Bhavnani SP. Digital Health: Opportunities and Challenges to Develop the Next-Generation Technology-Enabled Models of Cardiovascular Care. Methodist Debakey Cardiovasc J 2020;16(4):296–303.

60. Lee GA, Betz RR, Clements DH 3rd, et al. Proximal kyphosis after posterior spinal fusion in patients with idiopathic scoliosis. Spine 1999;24(8):795–9.

61. Glattes RC, Bridwell KH, Lenke LG, et al. Proximal junctional kyphosis in adult spinal deformity following long instrumented posterior spinal fusion: incidence, outcomes, and risk factor analysis. Spine 2005;30(14):1643–9.

62. Hostin R, McCarthy I, O'Brien M, et al. Incidence, mode, and location of acute proximal junctional failures after surgical treatment of adult spinal deformity. Spine 2013;38(12):1008–15.

63. Chan YFY, Wang P, Rogers L, et al. The Asthma Mobile Health Study, a large-scale clinical observational study using ResearchKit. Nat Biotechnol 2017;35(4):354–62.

64. Huckvale K, Venkatesh S, Christensen H. Toward clinical digital phenotyping: a timely opportunity to consider purpose, quality, and safety. NPJ Digit Med 2019;2:88.

65. Huckvale K, Torous J, Larsen ME. Assessment of the data sharing and privacy practices of smartphone apps for depression and smoking cessation. JAMA Netw Open 2019;2(4):e192542.

66. Abdolkhani R, Gray K, Borda A, et al. Patient-generated health data management and quality challenges in remote patient monitoring. JAMIA Open 2019;2(4):471–8.

Spinal Cord Injury
Emerging Technologies

Andrew M. Hersh, AB[a], Carly Weber-Levine, MS[a], Kelly Jiang, MS[a],
Nicholas Theodore, MS, MD[a,b],*

KEYWORDS

• Spine • SCI • Trauma • Injury • Ultrasound • CSF • Stem cell

KEY POINTS

• The primary treatments for spinal cord injury include elevation of mean arterial pressure above 85 mm Hg and decompressive surgery to reduce pressure on the cord.
• Stem cells, which can be injected at the site of injury via bioscaffolds, can promote regeneration of neurons.
• Advances in computer signaling and processing allow for the transmission of signals from the brain to a machine and onward to the spinal cord, bypassing the injured tracts and restoring control of motor movement.
• New techniques in ultrasound imaging allow for high-resolution imaging of spinal cord microvasculature and quantification of spinal cord perfusion, providing insights into injury progression and treatment response.
• Lumbar drains and smart catheters may improve functional outcomes by draining cerebrospinal fluid and reducing intrathecal pressure.

INTRODUCTION

Described in antiquity as a "medical condition that should not be treated," spinal cord injury (SCI) has undergone a dramatic revolution in management that has improved both survival and neurologic functions.[1] The pathophysiology of SCI involves a primary phase consisting of the initial mechanical injury, and a secondary phase of worsening damage characterized by ischemia, inflammation, excitotoxicity, and neuronal cell death. The secondary phase of injury can last several weeks.[2] Standard-of-care guidelines include decompressive surgery to relieve pressure on the spinal cord and augmentation of mean arterial pressure (MAP) to combat ischemia. Together, these treatments are aimed at improving spinal cord perfusion pressure (SCPP), calculated as the difference between MAP and intraspinal pressure (ISP).[3,4]

Unfortunately, no curative treatment exists for SCI, and although more people are surviving the initial event, outcomes remain poor. SCI can present significant functional limitations for people, including paraplegia, bowel and bladder incontinence, and chronic pain.[5] Substantial research is being conducted to explore therapeutic options that can mitigate against the secondary phase of injury or improve quality of life for people with chronic SCI. Recent laboratory experiments, case series, and clinical trials suggest that new improvements in SCI management may be on the horizon. Here, the authors review novel technologies that may improve outcomes after SCI.

DISCUSSION
Stem Cells

Stem cells have neuroregenerative properties and secrete cytokines, growth factors, and extracellular matrix proteins that mitigate damage from inflammation, combat neuronal apoptosis, and promote injury repair by inducing angiogenesis

[a] Department of Neurosurgery, Johns Hopkins University School of Medicine, 600 North Wolfe Street, Meyer 7-113, Baltimore, MD 21287, USA; [b] Orthopaedic Surgery & Biomedical Engineering, Department of Neurosurgery, Johns Hopkins University School of Medicine, Baltimore, MD, USA
* Corresponding author.
E-mail address: theodore@jhmi.edu
Twitter: @AndrewMHersh (A.M.H.); @kellyjjiang (K.J.); @DrNTheodore (N.T.)

Neurosurg Clin N Am 35 (2024) 243–251
https://doi.org/10.1016/j.nec.2023.10.001
1042-3680/24/© 2023 Elsevier Inc. All rights reserved.

and axonal growth.[6] Preclinical animal models have demonstrated successful delivery and survival of stem cells at the site of injury, as well as their ability to restore sensory signal pathways, reduce post-traumatic cavitation, and improve neurologic recovery.[6,7] For example, Zurita and colleagues showed recovery of somatosensory-evoked potentials and improvement in functional deficits in a porcine model after transplantation of bone marrow stromal cells into the spinal cord 3 months after injury.[8] The study illustrates the potential of stem cells to promote neuronal growth in patients outside of the initial acute window of injury.

Despite promising results in animal models and successful outcomes in treating other conditions such as hematological malignancies and burns, stem cell therapy for SCI remains controversial, and high-quality randomized studies are lacking.[9] A 2016 phase III trial of 16 patients demonstrated neurologic improvement in only two patients following a single injection of mesenchymal stem cells.[10] Challenges with stem cell therapy include limited survival due to immunologic attack from host cells, unfavorable inflammatory environments, and insufficient cell quantities.[10,11] A meta-analysis of 62 clinical trials of stem cell therapy in SCI documented improvement in the American Spinal Injury Association (ASIA) Impairment Scale grade by at least 1 point in half of the participants; however, concerning side effects included neuropathic pain, muscle spasms, and emesis. Furthermore, most clinical trials were single-arm studies with small sample sizes.[12] Tumorigenesis from stem cell proliferation and genetic instability is a concerning adverse event that is uncommon but has been reported after cell transplantation for SCI.[13,14]

Successful regenerative therapy will likely depend not only on the injection of stem cells at the site of injury but also on new technologies designed to improve the survival rate of stem cells while limiting their side effects. Optogenetics has been explored to control stem cell activation and to improve their neural connections with neighboring spinal cord cells. Clustered regularly interspaced short palindromic repeats (CRISPR), or CRISPR technology, has been proposed as a way to select stem cell phenotypes with improved survival and decreased immunologic rejection.[15] More recently, 3D-printed implants and scaffolds have emerged as delivery vectors to promote stem cell growth and survival; these tools can be customized to individual injuries, described in further detail below.[16] Stem cell-loaded bioreactors have also been shown to improve outcomes after myocardial infarction, with the bioreactor providing a protected space against immunologic attack, and may similarly be applied to SCI.[17] Successful applications of stem cell therapy for patients with SCI may require a combination of methods to improve delivery, stem cell survival, and functional recovery.

Scaffolds

Biocompatible scaffolds, also called *bioscaffolds*, are structures intended to promote healing of the injured spinal cord and regenerate neurons and axons. Inflammation during the secondary phase of SCI activates astrocytes and fibroblasts to remodel the extracellular matrix and form a glial scar, which creates a physical and chemical barrier to axonal regrowth. In addition, a cavity or cyst can form at the injury site. Neuroregenerative strategies seek to restore functional tissue and neuronal connections across the injury site to improve function. Schwann cells are neuroprotective and can be implanted at the injury site to promote axonal regrowth, whereas stem cells can be induced to differentiate into neuronal tissue. Similarly, astrocyte precursors are under investigation for their ability to treat glial scars and promote axonal regeneration.[18] Chondroitinase treatments and other enzymes can also be used to digest the glial scar, whereas the iron chelator deferoxamine can prevent its formation.[16]

Delivery of these biomaterials requires careful fabrication of a polymer composite scaffold. Such scaffolds can be formed using natural materials, such as hyaluronic acid, collagen, and cellulose or synthetic materials, such as polyethylene glycol and polylactic acid.[18] The scaffolds can also be 3D-printed and constructed as hydrogels.[19] The design construct of the scaffold considers the constituent compounds' effects on inflammation, angiogenesis, cellular adhesion and proliferation, and neuronal growth.[19]

Preclinical models of scaffolds used as drug delivery vehicles or loaded with stem cells for the treatment of SCI have been shown to reduce cavitation, promote neuronal repair, and facilitate axonal growth.[20,21] Studies in large animal models have confirmed restoration of locomotor activity using scaffolds.[22,23] For example, Rao and colleagues treated monkeys after severe SCI with chitosan loaded with neurotrophin-3, a neurotrophin that stimulates neurogenesis, neuronal differentiation, and synaptic formation. The scaffold was designed to release the neurotrophin slowly over 14 weeks. The researchers found significant axonal regeneration, with motor axons growing across the scaffold into distal areas of the cord, and the monkeys demonstrated corresponding improvement in motor and sensory function.[23]

The first implantation of a bioresorbable polymer scaffold in a patient with SCI was reported in 2016, with the patient improving from ASIA A to ASIA C at the 3-month follow-up.[24] The scaffold is designed to provide structural support to the injured cord and promote natural repair processes and was further studied in a clinical trial of 16 patients. The trial resulted in improvement of the ASIA grade by at least 1 point in 7 of 16 treated patients at the 6-month follow-up, with continued improvements in ASIA grade among select patients at the 2-year follow-up. No adverse events were noted, and this trial has paved the way for larger randomized trials.[25,26]

Brain–Spine Interfaces and Exoskeletons

Brain–spine interfaces (BSIs) are designed to restore the functional connections between the brain and the spinal cord. The technology has advanced remarkably in recent years, with Lorach and colleagues describing a BSI that restored natural walking in a 38-year-old man with an incomplete injury at C5–C6. Their BSI consists of four principal components: (1) cortical implants placed over the sensorimotor cortex to record electrocorticographic signals, (2) spinal electrodes placed over the dorsal root entry zone in the lumbosacral spine, (3) a wearable processing unit to predict motor intentions from the electrocorticographic data and direct stimulation, and (4) an implantable pulse generator to stimulate the spinal electrodes (**Fig. 1**).[27] Continued advancements in BSIs are expected to improve their ease of use and broaden their applicability to people with SCI.

Brain–computer interfaces similarly map electrocorticographic signals but direct stimulation to corresponding muscle groups in an extremity of interest, such as the arm or leg. For example, Bouton and colleagues constructed a device that uses machine learning algorithms to decode signals from the motor cortex and direct stimulation of a patient's forearm muscles. Their system restored six different wrist and hand motions to a person with quadriplegia, recovering key functional movements, such as grasping and manipulating objects.[28]

Exoskeletons, which are wearable robotics designed to augment motor function, can serve myriad purposes—from supporting body weight while a person moves, to recreating a desired movement.[29,30] Benefits of the exoskeleton include its ability to support body weight, stabilize the person, and avoid the spinal implants requisite for BSIs; however, tradeoffs include their bulk and cost. Several US Food and Drug Administration (FDA)-approved exoskeletons are available for rehabilitation and personal mobility. Similar to the BSIs described above, new versions of exoskeletons incorporate cortical control, where electrical signals from the sensorimotor cortex are processed and translated into movements for execution by the motorized exoskeleton.[31] Rehabilitation with exoskeletons can promote plasticity and neurologic recovery of both motor control and somatic sensations in people with SCI.[32]

Spinal Cord Stimulation

In 1986, Barolat and colleagues published a case report of a patient with an incomplete C5 SCI who received epidural spinal cord stimulation for treatment of severe spasms, noting that the patient regained some lower extremity voluntary motor function.[33] Epidural electrical stimulation (EES) has since been investigated as a means of restoring ambulatory function in individuals with paraplegia and SCIs.[34] Unlike BSIs, EES implants do not receive cortical input regarding the person's intention to move. Consequently, they require a degree of fine-tuning and sequential testing of various stimulation amplitudes and frequencies to determine the optimal combinations for stimulating muscles to initiate a desired movement.[35] The signals are refined during the programming phase of the EES as the person attempts the intended movement. Electrophysiological mapping and electromyography can be used to guide electrode placement and to ensure adequate coverage of desired muscle groups.[36]

Although the exact biological mechanisms underlying EES are unknown, stimulation is believed to recruit residual neuronal circuits and previously inactive nerve connections while promoting the plasticity of motor units. This plasticity helps eventually recover voluntary movements—even in the absence of stimulation.[37,38] A subpopulation of excitatory interneurons activated by EES has recently been identified as essential for recovering ambulation after SCI, even though these excitatory interneurons are not required for movement before injury.[39] Future applications targeting these specific neuronal populations may enhance EES therapy.

Importantly, EES has also shown benefits in people with complete injuries.[36,38] Therefore, the initiation of EES early after injury, when the cord is believed to retain the greatest degree of plasticity, is believed to optimize outcomes.[34] Extensive rehabilitation is critical for improving outcomes with EES, and patients often require greater than 6 months of therapy as they retrain their body and muscles to walk.[35,37] The stimulating electrodes are connected to devices, such as a voice-controlled watch, designed to initiate

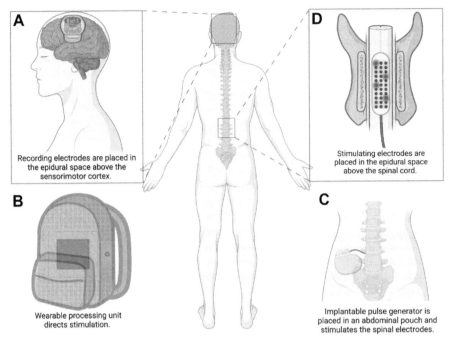

Fig. 1. A brain–spine interface, depicting (*A*) cortical signals from the brain relayed to (*B*) a wearable processing unit that interprets the signals and communicates with (*C*) an implantable pulse generator to stimulate (*D*) epidural electrodes over the spinal cord. (*Created with* BioRender.com.)

stimulation when the patient is ready to ambulate. A systematic review by Mansour and colleagues identified 184 people with SCI treated with EES, with nearly all individuals reporting some improvement in function.[40] However, further research is needed to identify the ideal stimulator settings, implantation site, and population most likely to benefit from this therapy.

Ultrasound

Ultrasound imaging offers a noninvasive, radiation-free means of imaging the injured spinal cord in real time and assessing morphologic and hemodynamic changes over time. The technology is more widely available and quicker than MRI, and it can be safely used in patients with metal fragments or shrapnel from a penetrating injury.[40] Increased echogenicity of the cord parenchyma, cyst formation, swelling, and compression of the subarachnoid space are visible on ultrasound. These morphologic changes correlate with the severity of the injury as assessed by the ASIA grade.[41] The bony anatomy of the spine typically presents a barrier to ultrasound imaging of the cord; however, removal of the bone during a decompressive laminectomy removes the acoustic shadowing, providing a window of opportunity in patients with SCI.[2]

Intraoperatively, standard B-mode ultrasound can be used to assess the extent of spinal cord decompression following a laminectomy, allowing surgeons to determine whether the laminectomy should be extended to relieve cord swelling and compression. The margins of the laminectomy site can be examined for residual compression by bony elements, and the rhythmic pulsatility of cerebrospinal fluid (CSF) can be assessed.[42] Chryssikos and colleagues studied intraoperative ultrasound in 51 SCI patients, reporting that 10% of patients underwent additional laminectomy to improve the decompression.[43] Another method of determining compression relies on shear-wave elastography, which is an ultrasound modality that measures stiffness by determining displacement from the propagation of shear waves across tissue.[44] Al-Habib and colleagues showed that spinal cord stiffness decreases following decompression in a study of 25 patients, although the application of elastography is not well studied in the SCI population.[45] Ultrasound can also identify the presence of intraparenchymal hemorrhage as a hyperechoic region within the cord parenchyma, and segmentation methods have been reported to extract quantitative characteristics.[46]

Ultrasound has additional value in monitoring spinal cord perfusion and determining the extent of ischemic changes. Contrast-enhanced ultrasound, which uses intravenous microbubbles to visualize blood flow, can illustrate hypoperfusion at the injury epicenter and monitor evolution over time, allowing clinicians to assess responses to therapy and/or need for more intensive therapy, such as further increases in MAP (**Fig. 2**).[47,48] Khaing and colleagues reported obtaining contrast-enhanced ultrasound imaging transcutaneously in a rodent SCI model 10 weeks after the initial injury, illustrating the potential use of ultrasound in a clinical setting.[49] However, contrast-enhanced ultrasound requires intravenous injections for imaging. New ultrasound modalities can provide detailed spatial resolution of blood flow in a noninvasive fashion. For example, Routkevitch and colleagues recently described an algorithm to extract quantitative measurements of blood flow over time across individual spinal cord vessels using noninvasive ultrasound recordings.[50]

Beyond its diagnostic potential, ultrasound can be used for therapeutic purposes. Focused ultrasound (FUS) technology produces energy from the concentration of ultrasound waves into a single point and includes high-intensity FUS (HIFUS) modalities with permanent ablation and low-intensity FUS (LIFUS) modalities with transient physiologic effects.[51,52] HIFUS may help relieve neuropathic pain from SCI by ablating targets in the thalamus, spinal cord, or peripheral nerves.[51] Protocols for disruption of the blood–spinal cord barrier in animal models using LIFUS have been reported, which may improve delivery of therapeutics and drugs to the site of injury.[53,54] LIFUS applied to the spinal cord has also been reported to modulate motor-evoked potentials in rodents, decrease inflammation, alleviate spasticity, and improve neuronal survival.[51,55,56] Research investigating FUS in the setting of SCI has been restricted to preclinical animal studies, but the positive outcomes pave the way for potential applications in humans.

Dural Decompression and Cerebrospinal Fluid Drainage

Swelling of the spinal cord obstructs normal flow of CSF and increases ISP, which can be measured using intradural pressure probes, which in turn reduce spinal cord perfusion. Durotomy, which decompresses the thecal sac and can restore the normal flow of CSF, has been reported to effectively decrease ISP to a greater extent than decompressive laminectomy alone. Duraplasty provides another means of alleviating dural compression and can be combined with durotomy. A study of 21 patients by Phang and colleagues showed that the combination of laminectomy and duraplasty caused greater reduction in ISP and improvement in SCPP compared with laminectomy alone. These researchers used a Codman pressure sensor (DePuy Synthes), inserted intradurally, to monitor ISP over time.[57] Aarabi and colleagues found that although most patients may achieve sufficient decompression with laminectomy alone, patients with severe swelling—which can be assessed with intraoperative ultrasound—may benefit from expansile duraplasty.[58]

CSF drainage (CSFD) has also been proposed to reduce ISP and improve perfusion.[59] CSFD has had an established role for decades in reducing spinal cord ischemia during surgical repair of thoracoabdominal aortic aneurysms; however, few studies have evaluated its efficacy for SCI. A recent trial enrolled 11 patients receiving lumbar drains after SCI and randomized them between a CSFD and control group while monitoring MAP and intrathecal pressure over a 5-day period. In that study, CSFD improved SCPP: The control group had a mean SCPP of 77 (4.5) mm Hg, whereas the group that received CSFD had a mean SCPP of 101 (6.3) mm Hg.[60] These findings

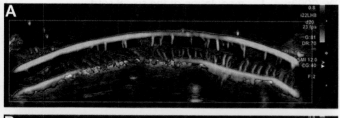
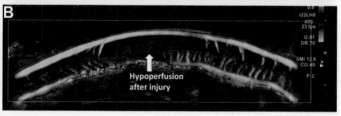

Hypoperfusion after injury

Fig. 2. (*A*) Pre-injury baseline ultrasound image of rodent microvasculature. (*B*) A decrease in perfusion is evident at the site of spinal cord injury.

suggest that CSFD is feasible and safe, but additional studies with larger cohorts are needed for validation of efficacy. CSFD can also allow for quantitative evaluation of biomarkers in the CSF that can track the progression of injury, including inflammatory biomarkers, such as interleukins and tumor necrosis factor alpha (TNF-α), as well as structural biomarkers, including neuron-specific enolase and glial fibrillary acidic protein. These biomarkers have been extensively studied as prognostic indicators of SCI, but require sampling from CSF and laboratory analysis, and therefore may not demonstrate acute changes.[61] However, lumbar catheters can be configured with optical fiber sensors for the detection of biomarkers in real-time, which work by detecting fluorescence and optical property changes of distinct biomarkers.[62] These catheters are not yet studied for SCI but have been reported for their application to traumatic brain injury and may be of use for clinicians performing CSFD.

Pharmacology

Medical management is an important adjunct to surgical treatment and warrants careful consideration after the initial injury. Methylprednisolone is one of the best-studied pharmacologic interventions for SCI, believed to improve outcomes through an anti-inflammatory effect.[63,64] However, most studies, including several randomized trials, have failed to demonstrate robust neurologic improvement with steroids and instead show an increase in severe complications.[65,66] Nonetheless, some still advocate for corticosteroids in select circumstances. For example, 2017 practice guidelines from AOSpine recommend 24-hour infusions for patients presenting within 8 hours but not those presenting later.[67]

Another important avenue for pharmacologic therapy is augmentation of MAP, which can be achieved with vasopressors, commonly dopamine, phenylephrine, or norepinephrine.[4] The administration of vasopressors is intended to improve SCPP and combat the ischemic processes of SCI. SCPP can be estimated as the difference between MAP and intrathecal pressure using intrathecal pressure monitors; however, ultrasound may eventually offer an alternative monitoring modality, as noted above.

There are several novel therapeutic agents that are being explored for SCI therapy. Polyphenols have been investigated to target the apoptotic pathways and reduce the inflammation characteristic of the secondary phase of injury.[68] For example, curcumin exerts anti-inflammatory effects, decreases oxidative stress, and can inhibit apoptotic pathways. A rat study showed that it improved ambulatory function after SCI.[69] Other anti-inflammatory molecules are being studied, such as minocycline, whose safety and feasibility were established in a clinical study of 52 patients, although the improvement in motor scores was not statistically significant.[70]

SUMMARY

Recent breakthroughs in scientific research, combined with advancements in technology and engineering, offer the promise of new SCI treatments. These therapeutics may assist patients in both the acute and chronic phases of injury. Some modalities, such as exoskeletons, ultrasound, and dural decompression, are already being incorporated into present-day clinical care. Others, such as stem cell treatments and bioscaffolds, require further research and randomized controlled trials to prove efficacy, which will undoubtedly unfold in the coming years.

CLINICS CARE POINTS

- Brain–spine interfaces are limited in availability and are invasive in nature; however, they offer the potential for people to regain some voluntary motor function by relaying cortical signals to the spinal cord.

- Epidural electrical stimulation produces long-term improvements in motor activity, even in people with complete spinal cord injuries.

- Ultrasound can be used intraoperatively to determine the adequacy of decompression; it can also provide insights into spinal cord perfusion.

- Focused ultrasound may play a role in neuromodulation of the spinal cord.

- Cerebrospinal fluid drainage using a standard lumbar catheter reduces intrathecal pressure, thereby increasing spinal cord perfusion pressure.

DISCLOSURES

N Theodore receives royalties from and owns stock in Globus Medical. He is a consultant for Globus Medical and has served on the scientific advisory board/other office for Globus Medical. The subject of this manuscript was deemed exempt from IRB approval.

REFERENCES

1. Van Middendorp JJ, Sanchez GM, Burridge AL. The Edwin Smith papyrus: a clinical reappraisal of the oldest known document on spinal injuries. Eur Spine J 2010;19(11):1815.

2. Tsehay Y, Weber-Levine C, Kim T, et al. Advances in Monitoring for Acute Spinal Cord Injury: A Narrative Review of Current Literature. Spine J 2022;0(0). https://doi.org/10.1016/J.SPINEE.2022.03.012.

3. Squair JW, Bélanger LM, Tsang A, et al. Empirical targets for acute hemodynamic management of individuals with spinal cord injury. Neurology 2019; 93(12):e1205–11.

4. Karsy M, Hawryluk G. Modern Medical Management of Spinal Cord Injury. Curr Neurol Neurosci Rep 2019;19(9):1–7.

5. Hersh AM, Davidar AD, Weber-Levine C, et al. Advancements in the treatment of traumatic spinal cord injury during military conflicts. Neurosurg Focus 2022;53(3). https://doi.org/10.3171/2022.6. FOCUS22262.

6. Cofano F, Boido M, Monticelli M, et al. Mesenchymal Stem Cells for Spinal Cord Injury: Current Options, Limitations, and Future of Cell Therapy. Int J Mol Sci 2019;20(11). https://doi.org/10.3390/IJMS20112698.

7. Gazdic M, Volarevic V, Randall Harrell C, et al. Stem Cells Therapy for Spinal Cord Injury. Int J Mol Sci 2018;19(4):1039.

8. Zurita M, Vaquero J, Bonilla C, et al. Functional recovery of chronic paraplegic pigs after autologous transplantation of bone marrow stromal cells. Transplantation 2008;86(6):845–53.

9. Goldring CEP, Duffy PA, Benvenisty N, et al. Assessing the safety of stem cell therapeutics. Cell Stem Cell 2011;8(6):618–28.

10. Oh SK, Choi KH, Yoo JY, et al. A Phase III Clinical Trial Showing Limited Efficacy of Autologous Mesenchymal Stem Cell Therapy for Spinal Cord Injury. Neurosurgery 2016;78(3):436–47.

11. Liau LL, Looi QH, Chia WC, et al. Treatment of spinal cord injury with mesenchymal stem cells. Cell Biosci 2020;10(1):1–17.

12. Shang Z, Wang M, Zhang B, et al. Clinical translation of stem cell therapy for spinal cord injury still premature: results from a single-arm meta-analysis based on 62 clinical trials. BMC Med 2022;20(1):1–19.

13. Ben-David U, Benvenisty N. The tumorigenicity of human embryonic and induced pluripotent stem cells. Nat Rev Cancer 2011;11(4):268–77.

14. Dlouhy BJ, Awe O, Rao RC, et al. Autograft-derived spinal cord mass following olfactory mucosal cell transplantation in a spinal cord injury patient: Case report. J Neurosurg Spine 2014;21(4):618–22.

15. Paschon V, Correia FF, Morena BC, et al. CRISPR, Prime Editing, Optogenetics, and DREADDs: New Therapeutic Approaches Provided by Emerging Technologies in the Treatment of Spinal Cord Injury. Mol Neurobiol 2020;57(4):2085–100.

16. Vogelaar CF, König B, Krafft S, et al. Pharmacological Suppression of CNS Scarring by Deferoxamine Reduces Lesion Volume and Increases Regeneration in an In Vitro Model for Astroglial-Fibrotic Scarring and in Rat Spinal Cord Injury In Vivo. PLoS One 2015;10(7).

17. Johnston PV, Hwang CW, Bogdan V, et al. Intravascular Stem Cell Bioreactor for Prevention of Adverse Remodeling After Myocardial Infarction. J Am Heart Assoc 2019;8(15).

18. Qu W, Chen B, Shu W, et al. Polymer-Based Scaffold Strategies for Spinal Cord Repair and Regeneration. Front Bioeng Biotechnol 2020;8. https://doi.org/10. 3389/FBIOE.2020.590549.

19. Sakiyama-Elbert S, Johnson PJ, Hodgetts SI, et al. Scaffolds to promote spinal cord regeneration. Handb Clin Neurol 2012;109:575–94.

20. Guest JD, Moore SW, Aimetti AA, et al. Internal decompression of the acutely contused spinal cord: Differential effects of irrigation only versus biodegradable scaffold implantation. Biomaterials 2018;185:284–300. Journal Article PG-284-300).

21. Koffler J, Zhu W, Qu X, et al. Biomimetic 3D-printed scaffolds for spinal cord injury repair. Nat Med 2019; 25(2):263–9.

22. Han S, Xiao Z, Li X, et al. Human placenta-derived mesenchymal stem cells loaded on linear ordered collagen scaffold improves functional recovery after completely transected spinal cord injury in canine. Sci China Life Sci 2018;61(1):2–13.

23. Rao JS, Zhao C, Zhang A, et al. NT3-chitosan enables de novo regeneration and functional recovery in monkeys after spinal cord injury. Proc Natl Acad Sci U S A 2018;115(24):E5595–604.

24. Theodore N, Hlubek R, Danielson J, et al. First Human Implantation of a Bioresorbable Polymer Scaffold for Acute Traumatic Spinal Cord Injury: A Clinical Pilot Study for Safety and Feasibility. Neurosurgery 2016;79(2):E305–12.

25. Kim KD, Lee KS, Coric D, et al. A study of probable benefit of a bioresorbable polymer scaffold for safety and neurological recovery in patients with complete thoracic spinal cord injury: 6-month results from the INSPIRE study. J Neurosurg Spine 2021; 34(5):808–17.

26. Kim KD, Lee KS, Coric D, et al. Acute Implantation of a Bioresorbable Polymer Scaffold in Patients With Complete Thoracic Spinal Cord Injury: 24-Month Follow-up From the INSPIRE Study. Neurosurgery 2022;90(6):668–75.

27. Lorach H, Galvez A, Spagnolo V, et al. Walking naturally after spinal cord injury using a brain–spine interface. Nature 2023;618(7963):126–33.

28. Bouton CE, Shaikhouni A, Annetta NV, et al. Restoring cortical control of functional movement in

a human with quadriplegia. Nature 2016;533(7602): 247–50.

29. Sale P, Russo EF, Russo M, et al. Effects on mobility training and de-adaptations in subjects with Spinal Cord Injury due to a Wearable Robot: A preliminary report. BMC Neurol 2016;16(1):1–8.

30. Hohl K, Giffhorn M, Jackson S, et al. A framework for clinical utilization of robotic exoskeletons in rehabilitation. J NeuroEng Rehabil 2022;19(1):1–8.

31. Benabid AL, Costecalde T, Eliseyev A, et al. An exoskeleton controlled by an epidural wireless brain–machine interface in a tetraplegic patient: a proof-of-concept demonstration. Lancet Neurol 2019;18(12):1112–22.

32. Donati ARC, Shokur S, Morya E, et al. Long-Term Training with a Brain-Machine Interface-Based Gait Protocol Induces Partial Neurological Recovery in Paraplegic Patients. Sci Rep 2016;6(1):1–16.

33. Barolat G, Myklebust JB, Wenninger W. Enhancement of voluntary motor function following spinal cord stimulation–case study. Appl Neurophysiol 1986;49(6):307–14.

34. Wagner FB, Mignardot JB, Le Goff-Mignardot CG, et al. Targeted neurotechnology restores walking in humans with spinal cord injury. Nature 2018; 563(7729):65–71.

35. Angeli CA, Boakye M, Morton RA, et al. Recovery of Over-Ground Walking after Chronic Motor Complete Spinal Cord Injury. N Engl J Med 2018;379(13): 1244–50.

36. Darrow D, Balser D, Netoff TI, et al. Epidural Spinal Cord Stimulation Facilitates Immediate Restoration of Dormant Motor and Autonomic Supraspinal Pathways after Chronic Neurologically Complete Spinal Cord Injury. J Neurotrauma 2019;36(15): 2325.

37. Gill ML, Grahn PJ, Calvert JS, et al. Neuromodulation of lumbosacral spinal networks enables independent stepping after complete paraplegia. Nat Med 2018;24(11):1677–82.

38. Rejc E, Angeli CA, Atkinson D, et al. Motor recovery after activity-based training with spinal cord epidural stimulation in a chronic motor complete paraplegic. Sci Rep 2017;7(1):1–12.

39. Kathe C, Skinnider MA, Hutson TH, et al. The neurons that restore walking after paralysis. Nature 2022;611(7936):540–7.

40. Stokum JA, Chryssikos T, Shea P, et al. Letter: Ultrasound in Traumatic Spinal Cord Injury: A Wide-Open Field. Neurosurgery 2022;90(4):E110–1.

41. Mirvis SE, Geisler FH. Intraoperative sonography of cervical spinal cord injury: results in 30 patients. Am J Neuroradiol 1990;11(4).

42. Ali DM, Harrop J, Sharan A, et al. Technical Aspects of Intra-Operative Ultrasound for Spinal Cord Injury and Myelopathy: A Practical Review. World Neurosurg 2023;170:206–18.

43. Chryssikos T, Stokum JA, Ahmed AK, et al. Surgical Decompression of Traumatic Cervical Spinal Cord Injury: A Pilot Study Comparing Real-Time Intraoperative Ultrasound After Laminectomy With Postoperative MRI and CT Myelography. Neurosurgery 2023; 92(2):353–62.

44. Hersh AM, Weber-Levine C, Jiang K, et al. Applications of elastography in operative neurosurgery: A systematic review. J Clin Neurosci 2022;104:18–28.

45. Al-Habib A, Alhothali W, Albakr A, et al. Effects of compressive lesions on intraoperative human spinal cord elasticity. J Neurosurg Spine 2021;1–10.

46. Malomo T, Allard Brown A, Bale K, et al. Quantifying Intraparenchymal Hemorrhage after Traumatic Spinal Cord Injury: A Review of Methodology. J Neurotrauma 2022;39(23–24):1603–35.

47. Khaing ZZ, Cates LN, DeWees DM, et al. Contrast-enhanced ultrasound to visualize hemodynamic changes after rodent spinal cord injury. J Neurosurg Spine 2018;29(3):306–13.

48. Weber-Levine C, Hersh AM, Jiang K, et al. Porcine Model of Spinal Cord Injury: A Systematic Review. Neurotrauma Rep 2022;3(1):352–68.

49. Khaing ZZ, Cates LN, Hyde JE, et al. Transcutaneous contrast-enhanced ultrasound imaging of the posttraumatic spinal cord. Spinal Cord 2020; 58(6):695–704.

50. Routkevitch D, Hersh AM, Kempski KM, et al. Flow-Morph: Morphological Segmentation of Ultrasound-Monitored Spinal Cord Microcirculation. IEEE Biomed Circuits Syst Conf 2022;2022:610.

51. Hwang BY, Mampre D, Ahmed AK, et al. Ultrasound in Traumatic Spinal Cord Injury: A Wide-Open Field. Neurosurgery 2021;89(3):372–82.

52. Hersh AM, Bhimreddy M, Weber-Levine C, et al. Applications of Focused Ultrasound for the Treatment of Glioblastoma: A New Frontier. Cancers 2022; 14(19).

53. Song Z, Ye Y, Zhang Z, et al. Noninvasive, targeted gene therapy for acute spinal cord injury using LIFU-mediated BDNF-loaded cationic nanobubble destruction. Biochem Biophys Res Commun 2018; 496(3):911–20.

54. Bhimreddy M, Routkevitch D, Hersh AM, et al. Disruption of the Blood-Spinal Cord Barrier using Low-Intensity Focused Ultrasound in a Rat Model. J Vis Exp 2023. 193.

55. Tsehay Y, Zeng Y, Weber-Levine C, et al. Low-Intensity Pulsed Ultrasound Neuromodulation of a Rodent's Spinal Cord Suppresses Motor Evoked Potentials. IEEE Trans Biomed Eng 2023;(7):70.

56. Liao YH, Chen MX, Chen SC, et al. Low-Intensity Focused Ultrasound Alleviates Spasticity and Increases Expression of the Neuronal K-Cl Cotransporter in the L4–L5 Sections of Rats Following Spinal Cord Injury. Front Cell Neurosci 2022;16: 882127.

57. Phang I, Werndle MC, Saadoun S, et al. Expansion Duroplasty Improves Intraspinal Pressure, Spinal Cord Perfusion Pressure, and Vascular Pressure Reactivity Index in Patients with Traumatic Spinal Cord Injury: Injured Spinal Cord Pressure Evaluation Study. J Neurotrauma 2015;32(12):865.

58. Aarabi B, Chixiang C, Simard JM, et al. Proposal of a Management Algorithm to Predict the Need for Expansion Duraplasty in American Spinal Injury Association Impairment Scale Grades A-C Traumatic Cervical Spinal Cord Injury Patients. J Neurotrauma 2022;39(23–24):1716–26.

59. Weber-Levine C, Judy BF, Hersh AM, et al. Multimodal interventions to optimize spinal cord perfusion in patients with acute traumatic spinal cord injuries: a systematic review. J Neurosurg Spine 2022;37(5):729–39.

60. Theodore N, Martirosyan N, Hersh AM, et al. Cerebrospinal Fluid Drainage in Patients with Acute Spinal Cord Injury: A Multi-Center Randomized Controlled Trial. World Neurosurg 2023. https://doi.org/10.1016/j.wneu.2023.06.078.

61. Albayar AA, Roche A, Swiatkowski P, et al. Biomarkers in Spinal Cord Injury: Prognostic Insights and Future Potentials. Front Neurol 2019;10(JAN):27.

62. Zhang Y, Hu Y, Liu Q, et al. Multiplexed optical fiber sensors for dynamic brain monitoring. Matter 2022; 5(11):3947–76.

63. Dumont RJ, Verma S, Okonkwo DO, et al. Acute spinal cord injury, part II: contemporary pharmacotherapy. Clin Neuropharmacol 2001;24(5):265–79.

64. Hurlbert RJ, Hadley MN, Walters BC, et al. Pharmacological therapy for acute spinal cord injury. Neurosurgery 2015;76(Suppl 1):S71–83.

65. Evaniew N, Noonan VK, Fallah N, et al. Methylprednisolone for the Treatment of Patients with Acute Spinal Cord Injuries: A Propensity Score-Matched Cohort Study from a Canadian Multi-Center Spinal Cord Injury Registry. J Neurotrauma 2015;32(21): 1674.

66. Hurlbert RJ. Methylprednisolone for the treatment of acute spinal cord injury: point. Neurosurgery 2014; 61(Suppl 1):32–5.

67. Fehlings MG, Wilson JR, Tetreault LA, et al. A Clinical Practice Guideline for the Management of Patients With Acute Spinal Cord Injury: Recommendations on the Use of Methylprednisolone Sodium Succinate. Global Spine J 2017;7(3 Suppl): 203S–11S.

68. Abbaszadeh F, Fakhri S, Khan H. Targeting apoptosis and autophagy following spinal cord injury: Therapeutic approaches to polyphenols and candidate phytochemicals. Pharmacol Res 2020; 160.

69. Gokce EC, Kahveci R, Gokce A, et al. Curcumin Attenuates Inflammation, Oxidative Stress, and Ultrastructural Damage Induced by Spinal Cord Ischemia–Reperfusion Injury in Rats. J Stroke Cerebrovasc Dis 2016;25(5):1196–207.

70. Casha S, Zygun D, McGowan MD, et al. Results of a phase II placebo-controlled randomized trial of minocycline in acute spinal cord injury. Brain 2012; 135(Pt 4):1224–36.

Artificial Intelligence in Spine Surgery

Justin K. Scheer, MD*, Christopher P. Ames, MD

KEYWORDS

- Artificial intelligence • Machine learning • Predictive modeling • Adult spinal deformity • Scoliosis
- Outcomes • Complications

KEY POINTS

- There is currently an explosion of data in healthcare allowing for the creation of artificial intelligence and machine learning algorithms.
- Artificial intelligence in spine surgery is only just beginning with the potential to predict patient specific postoperative complications, patient reported outcome metrics (PROMs), and costs to aid in resource allocation and bundled payments.
- Future data that should be included in artificial intelligence algorithms are the patients' biological features such as, objective physical metrics, biological clocks, biomarkers, and "omics" fields.

INTRODUCTION

There is a digital revolution occurring in the healthcare industry as the amount and type of data being generated continues to explode.[1] Specifically in medicine, artificial intelligence (AI) and machine learning (ML) have begun to transform the field of spine surgery as surgical outcomes databases continue to grow allowing for such types of analyses to be conducted.[2] By implementing AI/ML within spine surgery, the ability to detect what were previously undiscoverable patterns in data now become discoverable having the potential to enhance our predictive abilities unlike anything seen before, thus resulting widespread implications for the field as whole. Spine surgery is a complex field in which many different variables contribute to a patient's surgical outcome. Up until now, surgeons have been relying on data from the literature to inform treatment decision making, patient discussions, complication profiles, and potential for clinical success. However, these data tend to be based on population data which are heterogenous and lumped into averages by the use of traditional statistical methods. It is not patient specific, and thus, has serious limitations when attempting to predict a patient's outcome. Although this type of traditional analyses has been critical to advancing the field and has yielded clinical benefit, a paradigm shift is occurring now with AI/ML. Surgeons can now use these complex and sophisticated approaches to data to help tailor their practices for individual patient outcome prediction and further improve the chances of surgical success. This review will expand on AI/AL methodology and discuss how it has been applied to adult spinal deformity (ASD) surgery.

METHODOLOGY OF PREDICTIVE MODELING AND ARTIFICIAL INTELLIGENCE/MACHINE LEARNING

In order to better appreciate how AI and ML are currently being applied in spine surgery, it is critical to understand some of their basic features and how these types of complex analyses differ from more historical/traditional statistics. It is important to note that statistical models currently have and will continue to have an important role in surgical outcomes research. These methods, including linear and logistic regressions, have provided significant clinical applicability and insight

Department of Neurological Surgery, University of California, San Francisco, CA, USA
* Corresponding author. Department of Neurological Surgery, University of California, San Francisco 505 Parnassus Ave, Room M779, San Francisco, CA 94143.
E-mail address: jks2243@cumc.columbia.edu

Neurosurg Clin N Am 35 (2024) 253–262
https://doi.org/10.1016/j.nec.2023.11.001
1042-3680/24/© 2023 Elsevier Inc. All rights reserved.

into specific variables that help with risk prediction or clinical score creation; however, there are several specific factors regarding their applications when compared to AI or ML. Above all, traditional statistical models are designed to describe the relationship between the data and an outcome variable, therefore elucidating different relationships between the chosen variables and to test different a priori hypotheses. In general, they do not account for any individual patient changes and they produce odds/hazard ratios for any given clinical variable of interest for a certain cohort. Furthermore, these types of models are bound by many assumptions and must meet certain criteria for their applicability. These limitations inherently make them not ideal for use in developing patient specific predictive models.[3]

On contrary predictive analytical algorithms, specifically AI and ML, are designed to identify patterns in the data that allow for accurate predictions without the need for a hypothesis.[3–5] These methods are extremely useful for many reasons, one of which is their ability to process an extremely large amount of data with many heterogenous variables to make highly accurate and repeatable predictions. Although statistical models lack predictive ability and patient specificity, they are generally easy to both interpret and for other researchers to duplicate as they are quite transparent. AI and ML algorithms have a greater utility and are much more powerful for prediction, but at the cost of reduced transparency, the "black box", and can be difficult to interpret or replicate.[4,5] Despite this, current predictive analytics methods using AI or ML allow for the creation of accurate, patient specific, predictive models that can aid in clinical decision making.

When categorizing the current complex predictive analytics models, AI is at the top so to speak in terms of complexity and predictive abilities (**Fig. 1**). AI embodies the notion of computer algorithms attempting to simulate human intelligence by its ability to process large amounts of information and learn based on this data to make decisions and change behavior in areas such as speech recognition and visual perception.[4,5] AI itself consists of numerous computational techniques to accomplish this goal with the most relevant and common technique being ML. ML is a subset of AI that can process a huge amount of data, learn and adapt to new data introduced, and provide powerful and accurate predictions.[2] For all of these advanced modeling techniques, a "training dataset" is first used to create the initial algorithms on a given dataset. Ideally the dataset is very large and heterogenous; the larger the better.[3] The algorithms determine mathematical

relationships within the data without the influence of humans. This removes any selection bias of variables and with its ability to process an extraordinary amount of data, new data pattens/relationships can be identified that were not readily apparent or even intuitive before. After the algorithms have been trained, they are then "tested" on a different dataset to evaluate their accuracy and reliability.[3] The test set results are what tend to be reported and provide some insight into how well the model is performing to aid in determining if it is ready for deployment. Deployment refers to actually using the final model from the tested dataset on new data and then making decisions based on these results in realtime.[3] When training and testing algorithms, generally the dataset used is split for each function respectively either in a 70:30 or 80:20 split.[3,6] This implies 70% of the dataset is used for training while the remaining 30% is used for testing. When the models are being trained, there is a significant iterative process in which a variety of different potential models are evaluated for efficacy using a technique called cross-validation. Cross-validation refers to the training data being randomly and repeatedly partitioned. This results in a portion of the actual training data becoming a "validation set", in order to serve a similar purpose to the test set and allow for model optimization. **Fig. 2** represents a summary of this process. Once model performance is deemed sufficient on the test set, it is then be deployed. On the order of complexity, next is deep learning (see **Fig. 1**) that uses artificial neural networks that simulate neurons in the brain to also process large amounts of data and find important patterns. Following this would then be advanced predictive analytics algorithms, some of which include decision tree analysis, K-nearest neighbor, and Naïve Bayes.[3] It is beyond the scope of this review to discuss each method in detail; however, these algorithms can provide predictive models on their own or they can be incorporated in to larger complex analyses using multiple models and be included in ML and AI algorithms.

PREDICTIVE MODELING, ARTIFICIAL INTELLIGENCE AND MACHINE LEARNING IN ADULT SPINAL DEFORMITY

ASD surgery happens to be the subset of spine surgery that allows for the unique application of predictive modeling due to the extensive variability in ASD patients themselves, their clinical presentation, and the many factors that contribute to ASD surgical outcomes. Moreover, ASD patients tend to be frail[7] and surgical correction is often associated with high complication rates.[8] ASD surgical

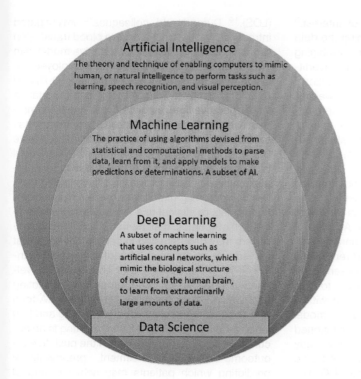

Fig. 1. Visual representation of artificial intelligence and its corresponding subsets. Data science can be seen as traversing all domains, as these are all commonly employed techniques in data science and analytics.[4]. (*From* Joshi RS, Haddad AF, Lau D, Ames CP. Artificial Intelligence for Adult Spinal Deformity. Neurospine. Dec 2019;16(4):686-694. https://doi.org/10.14245/ns.1938414.207.)

outcomes research was one of the first fields to adopt and explore this approach and now has grown to AI and ML with many other fields in spine surgery also applying these complex analytical methods.

The first few predictive models did not directly employ AI or ML but rather advanced predictive analytics, specifically decision tree analysis for complication prediction.[9–12] Briefly, these algorithms create classification trees allowing for

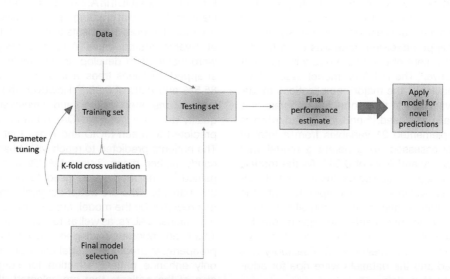

Fig. 2. Flow chart demonstrating the general process of training, validating, and testing utilized during the development of machine learning models.[6]. (*From* Joshi and colleagues, State-of-the-art reviews predictive modeling in adult spinal deformity: applications of advanced analytics,[6] Spine Deformity, with permission under the Creative Commons Attribution 4.0 International License, http://creativecommons.org/licenses/by/4.0/, with no changes made.)

prediction of an outcome variable of interest.[3] They can be optimized by bootstrapping the data to make it more generalizable or combining different trees into ensembles to minimize overfitting and to improve the accuracy of prediction.[3] The first predictive model in ASD surgery was reported by Scheer and colleagues and the International Spine Study Group (ISSG) to predict proximal junctional failure (PJF) or clinically significant proximal junctional kyphosis (PJK) within 2-yerars postoperative.[11] The authors used an ensemble of decisions trees and bootstrapped models in a cohort of 510 ASD patients.[11] The overall accuracy of the final model was 86% with area under the curve (AUC) of 0.89. An AUC is calculated from a receiver operator characteristic (ROC) curve for a binary outcome and represents the model's ability to distinguish between the 2 outcome variables.[3] An AUC closer to the maximum of 1 implies perfect prediction with a value of 0.5 implying a 50/50 chance of the model predicting the outcome.[3] The earlier mentioned PJF/PJK model was more of a feasibility study as to whether a model of this nature could be created with reasonable accuracy and AUC. The data were of sufficient amount and quality and thus, more models where then created. Following the PJK/PJF model, Scheer and colleagues created another model using similar techniques for 557 patients to predict major intraoperative or perioperative complications. The accuracy was 87% with an AUC of 0.89[12] further validating the feasibility for large spine study groups with prospective databases to create accurate predictive models. To augment the major complications model, another model using the similar techniques of bootstrapped decision trees was used to predict development of pseudarthrosis within 2-year postoperative.[9] The PJK/PJF model used a total of 13 variables,[11] the major complications model used 20 variables in the model after 45 variables were initially assessed,[12] and the pseudarthrosis model implemented 21 variables from a total of 82 initially assessed, to generate a model with 91% accuracy and AUC of 0.94.[9] As the models became more advanced so did the number of variables being evaluated and incorporated into the model. As complications play a critical role in the clinical outcomes of patients undergoing complex ASD surgery, it is no surprise these were the types of early predictive models in ASD. Feasibility was established and the datasets were ripe for additional types of models.

The next set of models were expanded from predicting postoperative complications to predicting intraoperative and perioperative variables such as transfusion requirements[13] and length of stay (LOS).[14] Durand and colleagues[13] investigated intraoperative and postoperative blood transfusion requirements and created a predictive model with 1029 ASD patients. The authors also employed decision tree analyses resulting in AUCs of 0.79 and 0.85.[13] The model variables of most importance were operative time, surgical invasiveness, hematocrit, weight, and age resulting in a simple and easy to implement model to help predict postoperative transfusions following ASD surgery.[13] This model is another good example of how these more complex analyses can improve the clinical care of patients undergoing high risk surgeries. Not only are the models of clinical use, but building models to predict outcomes that hospitals and third-party payers may be interested in can potentially assist in resource allocation and bundled payment planning. Therefore, Safaee and colleagues[14] developed a generalized linear model for predicting LOS within 2 days following ASD surgery. A total of 653 patients were included for training and 240 independent patients for testing resulting in an accuracy of 75.4%.[14] Similarly, with the push toward outcome-based reimbursement, preoperatively predicting which patients may achieve surgical success could significantly aid in patient selection, resource utilization, and paired surgical decision making with the surgeon and patient.

Patient reported outcome metrics (PROMs) are factored into the surgical decision making of the surgeon and thus became the subject of predictive modeling such as reaching the minimally important clinical difference (MCID) for the Oswestry Disability Index (ODI) in ASD patients.[10] Oh and colleagues[15] looked at creating a preoperative predictive model to predict patients achieving ODI MCID at 2-years postoperative. A total of 234 patients were included to develop an ensemble of bootstrapped decisions trees yielding an accuracy of 85.5% and AUC of 0.96.[15] However, the authors took it one step further and investigated the quality-adjusted life years (QALYs) of the patients predicted to reach MCID and those that did not. The patients predicted to reach MCID had significantly higher mean 2-year QALYs and QALYs gained.[15] The model was used to demonstrate that patients, who are better surgical candidates, as predicted by the model, are also more likely to have higher QALYs, as well as to gain more QALYs. This is an important finding as it highlights how a preoperative predictive model can potentially not only enhance patient selection for surgery but also of the patients that are selected, they can possibly have greater overall improvement in their health via the QALY analysis.

As the knowledge base and comfort of surgeons and researchers increased with every new predictive modeling paper, so did the techniques. Complex models using ML and AI were born. In addition, over this time, more high-quality data had been collected yielding larger datasets primed for more complex types of analyses. The ISSG and the European spine study group (ESSG) combined both of their high-quality datasets allowing AI and ML to create novel and more robust clinically applicable predictive models. These datasets are not only large and are very granular but span multiple countries, states, institutions, with many spine surgeons. To expand on the earlier PROM predictive models using the combined database, Ames and colleagues[16] conducted a very extensive analysis on predicting PROMs. The model used 570 ASD patients to predict the likelihood of reaching postoperative MCID in three major PROMs that included ODI, Scoliosis Research Society – 22 (SRS-22), and Medical Short Form – 36 (SF-36) at one- and 2-year follow-up.[16] This study was likely the most advanced and comprehensive at the time as it utilized 75 input variables for model development and evaluated the performance of eight different ML algorithms to optimize MCID prediction.[16] Moreover, each algorithm was trained at four specific time points: preoperative, immediate postoperative, 1-year follow-up, and at 2-year follow-up. The performances of the different models were evaluated via the mean average error (MAE) between them with the final model selection based on minimizing MAE and maximizing the goodness of fit via $R2$ values.[16] The MAE values between the models ranged from 8% to 15%, which suggests successful model creation and very accurate prediction ability.[16] It was interesting that neither the surgeon nor the institution were important factors in the models allowing for even more generalizability for other surgeons to employ these models.[16] Following the success of the earlier mentioned study, the PROM concept was expanded to attempt predicting individual patient responses to the PROMs using ML. Again, Ames and colleagues[17] with the ISSG/ESSG developed 6 different ML algorithms with 150 patient variables that successfully predicted individual patient answers to each of the SRS-22 questions, with AUC ranging from 0.57 to 0.87. This study is significant for a few reasons, first of which is the large amount of input variables. Using 150 variables is a long way from the 13 to 20 input variables initially used in the earlier models.[9,11] Second, the authors were able to achieve a very high level of granularity in the predictive model by predicting individual responses to the questions versus binary outcomes of developing a complication or not. Third, 1 of the major goals of accurate and reliable predictive

models is to eventually generate patient-specific predictions for personalized spine care. The ability to predict MCID at 1 or 2-years postop or to predict the individual patient responses to PROMs is a significant step toward individualized patient spine care. These algorithms are not designed to replace the surgeon by any means, but rather allow surgeons to corroborate their clinical recommendations to patients with sound data and models to aid in precision medicine by ultimately maximizing patient safety while improving surgical success.

The ISSG and ESSG continued their combined effort and developed more complex ML models for complications as the complication rates in ASD surgery remains high. Both patients and surgeons have concern over complication development, and thus, there is always a continued effort to minimize complications for these more technically challenging surgeries. The earlier models for complication prediction were valid and provided some clinical benefit; however, they were more of a proof-of-concept analysis and the data were not as robust. With the combined ISSG/ESSG data, the authors approached predicting postoperative complications again but with more advanced analytics. Pellise and colleagues[18] developed ML algorithms for predicting major complications, hospital readmission, and unplanned reoperations. A total of 105 clinical and radiographic variables were implemented with a large cohort of 1612 prospectively collected patients for model development.[18] The models were a successful having AUCs ranging from 0.67 to 0.92.[18] These models more closely resemble the type that could be employed in the clinical setting and aid in patient selection and shared surgical decision making between the surgeon and patient. The models would be continuously updated and predictions adjusted as new data are entered allowing for constant improvement.

In addition to prediction of postoperative complications and PROMs, preoperative patient classification can be an excellent adjunct in surgical planning and prognostication.[19,20] However, both the radiographic and clinical presentations for ASD patients are very heterogeneous resulting in current classification system being limited in nature. The gold standard for ASD classification systems have relied solely on radiographic features which do not account for any clinical patient factors.[19,20] This situation is ideal for AI as it can analyze hundreds of variables, infinitely more than any human has the capacity or time for, and developed an objective, data-driven classification system. This is just what Ames and colleagues[21] accomplished with unsupervised learning AI algorithms. The approach of unsupervised learning is different than the prior models described which were supervised. The data in supervised models are considered "labeled" by defining input and output variables a priori.[3] In the prior models for example, patient factors were defined as input variables and complication development would be defined as an output. The model then finds data patterns that link the input to the output variables. In unsupervised learning models, the data are not defined and there is no direct outcome variable(s) designated by the user. This approach to AI/ML can be very powerful as the algorithm is free to discern any patterns that may exist inherent to the data itself resulting in connections/predictions that may not have been apparent in the beginning. Ames and colleagues included 570 ASD patients and employed AI hierarchical clustering to identify different populations of ASD patients based on the data alone in order to better classify them.[21] Many variables were incorporated into the model that included patient data, surgical characteristics, PROM data, and patient demographic information. This was the most comprehensive classification attempt at the time. The results were very interesting and demonstrated 3 distinct ASD patient clusters: 1) young patients with coronal deformity, 2) older patients with high incidence of prior spine surgery, and 3) older patients with low incidence of prior spine surgery (**Fig. 3**). Furthermore, each of these new clusters was unique and displayed their own distinct outcomes profiles. This was the first time that unsupervised AI was used to classify patients and is an excellent example of how this type of analysis can offer incredible granularity and accuracy. It once again demonstrates the power of AI in clinical care and its potential to greatly improve surgical outcomes.

The earlier studies represented important milestones in ASD predictive modeling and have now expanded to benchmarking. Benchmarking is a method of process-improvement and can aid in the improvement of surgical outcomes. However, benchmarking generally employs averages or a ranking system and there is no gold standard method to do this. ML can potentially standardize this area of medicine by accurately predicting a certain benchmark that is site specific based on its own patient population and resources. Joshi and colleagues published preliminary data from the ISSG evaluating predictive models for PJF/PJK benchmarking.[6] Predictive models were created to determine site-specific PJK/PJF rates. The actual rates at each site were then compared to their predicted rate, rather than an overall average rate across all sites, in order to establish

a site-specific evaluation of their performance (**Fig. 4**). Thus, some sites were above or below their predicted rate. This was also done for pseudarthrosis with similar findings. Some sites were below the overall average indicating good performance on traditional metrics but above their predicted rate indicating poor site-specific performance. These early studies into using predictive modeling for benchmarking offer promise for future use to allow for more accurate surgeon and center specific performance evaluations.

And lastly, predictive modeling can be used for cost analyses, which could not only benefit hospital systems but also third-party payers. Within ASD surgery, Ames and colleagues[22] developed additional models with similar methodology to predict which patients may succumb to catastrophic costs following surgery at 90-days and 2-year postoperative. Using advanced random forest models and regression trees, the models reported R2 values ranging from 56% to 57% for 90-day direct cost, and 29% to 35% for 2-year direct cost prediction.[22] It is important to note that these methods may not be as complex as the other models for complication and cluster prediction, however the benefit is that these have both great prediction and are more transparent resulting in easier interpretations of the results. This is another important study to highlight that predictive modeling not only can be employed for surgical success metrics and complication reduction, but also potentially to help determine bundled payments and resource allocation for stakeholders outside of the clinical setting, thus, having the potential to make system wide improvement to care and resource utilization.

FUTURE DIRECTIONS

It is clear from the earlier discussions of predictive modeling and AI/ML in ASD surgery that these techniques offer great promise in advancing patient specific treatment plans while also improving the safety of surgery. However, these models rely on patient demographics, radiographic markers, PROMs, and surgical variables to make their predictions. They are all lacking the inherent biology/physical function of the patient, which would include specific aspects of the patients' objective physical abilities, innate physiology, genetics, and "omics" (transcriptomics, genomics, proteomics, metabolomics, etc).[23] Connected to all of these biological systems is the concept of frailty. Frailty is the phenotypic difference between chronologic age and physiologic age which is influenced by genetics and epigenetics.[23] It has been demonstrated repeatedly that frail patients are

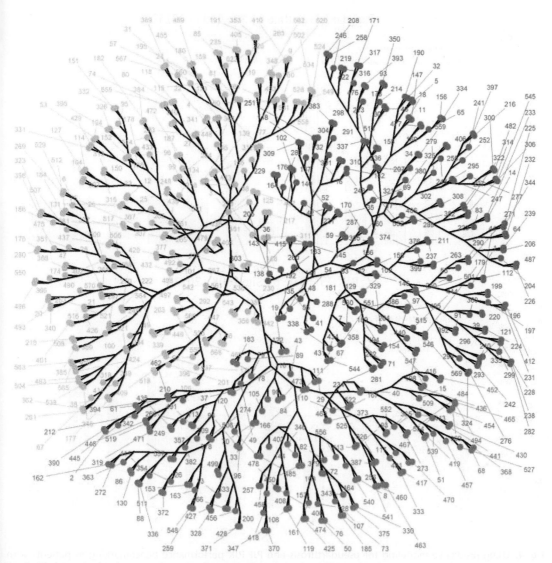

Fig. 3. Phylogenic dendrogram from application of unsupervised hierarchical clustering to patient parameters. Each dot represents a patient of the sample and colors represent the portions of the dendrogram in each of the 3 patient clusters. Blue represents young coronal patients (YC), yellow old revision patients (ORev) and gray old first time (OPrim). Patients with similar characteristics are placed closer to the center of each cluster, while being closer to the borders present observations with greater intra-cluster and lower inter-cluster variability.[21]. (*From* Ames and colleagues Artificial Intelligence Based Hierarchical Clustering of Patient Types and Intervention Categories in Adult Spinal Deformity Surgery: Toward a New Classification Scheme that Predicts Quality and Value,[21] Spine, with permission and no changes made.)

more likely to have worse postoperative outcomes.[7] Frailty has been traditionally defined as a clinical phenotype, including sarcopenia, medical comorbidities, and reduced physical function (walking speeds and grip strength). Therefore including the biological mechanisms behind the clinical presentation of frailty could be additional variables to add into the predictive models potentially making them more accurate and patient specific.[23] Moreover, adding in specific objective

physical metrics such as walking speeds can also add valuable data to the models that go beyond the patient's subjective feelings depicted on PROMs to more concrete and measurable data.

In addition to biologically characterizing the frailty phenotype and adding in objective physical metrics to the models, the overall physiology may have an impact on the patients' ability to not only tolerate a large surgery but also to potentially

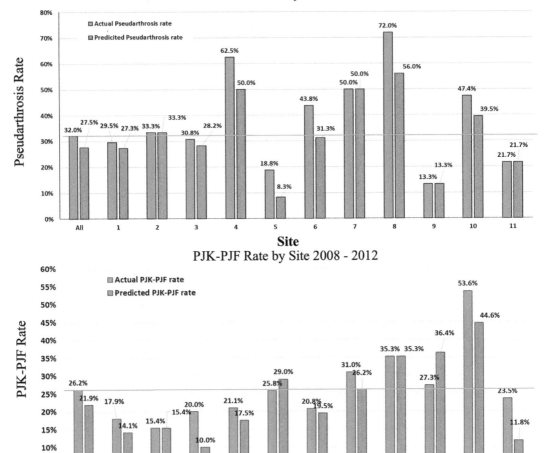

Fig. 4. Using predictive modeling for pseudarthrosis and PJF-PJK performance benchmarking in patients with minimum 2-year follow-up. Actual rates for pseudarthrosis and PJF-PJK are compared to site-specific predicted rates. The green line indicates average overall complication rate across all sites. Even though sites may have rates higher than the overall average, it is important to consider their higher predicted rates as well. Several sites demonstrated actual rates below the overall average but were still shown to be underperforming based on their predicted rates, while a couple showed actual rates higher than the average but lower than their predicted rates indicating higher performance.[6] (*From* Joshi and colleagues, State-of-the-art reviews predictive modeling in adult spinal deformity: applications of advanced analytics,[6] Spine Deformity, with permission under the Creative Commons Attribution 4.0 International License, http://creativecommons.org/licenses/by/4.0/, with no changes made.)

form a solid fusion, have proper wound healing, and even to incur postoperative complications. A study by Safaee and colleagues investigated telomere length and postoperative complications following ASD surgery and found that genetic age was significantly associated with the risk of complications despite no significant difference in chronologic age.[24] This is a key finding as it was the first time in spine surgery that a patient's

biology was directly linked to postsurgical complications indicating that the prior predictive models have been missing this vital information when attempting to accurately predict postoperative outcomes. It has become commonplace within the basic sciences disciples to include some type of genetic analysis; however, these have not yet permeated into surgical outcomes studies let alone predictive modeling. More recently, stemming from genetics, new fields have emerged that include transcriptomics, proteomics, and metabolomics[25]; the end of the biological chain of events. Metabolomics refers to the study of metabolites within the human body.[26,27] These metabolites can play critical roles in physiopathological processes as they regulate cellular activity and mediate biological function with approximately 18,500 quantified metabolites thus far.[27,28] The field of metabolomics investigates many of these metabolites and is highly sensitive in being able to discover normal and abnormal mechanisms of the body through subtle biological changes.[27] Therefore metabolomics can provide a "big-picture" overview of the patient and as well as significantly add to the current AI/ML algorithms.[23] The addition of biological data from biological clocks, genetics, and the "omics" fields could potentially advance the AI/ML algorithms at an incredible pace.

CLINIC CARE POINTS

- Artificial intelligence (AI) and Machine Learning (ML) are complex computational techniques that allow for powerful prediction of surgical outcomes
- Large and high-quality datasets are necessary to employ AI/ML techniques for accurate prediction
- Future models will include patients' biological data to increase the predictive power of the algorithms
- Point of care AI/ML predictive models will become more prevalent in the future as the datasets become larger and more accessible

DISCLOSURE

There are no financial conflicts of interest related to this article.

REFERENCES

1. Subrahmanya SVG, Shetty DK, Patil V, et al. The role of data science in healthcare advancements: applications, benefits, and future prospects. Ir J Med Sci 2022;191(4):1473–83.
2. Lee NJ, Lombardi JM, Lehman RA. Artificial Intelligence and Machine Learning Applications in Spine Surgery. Internet J Spine Surg 2023;17(S1):S18–25.
3. Abbott D. Applied predictive analytics : principles and techniques for the professional data analyst. 1st edition. John Wiley & Sons, Inc.; 2014. p. 427.
4. Joshi RS, Haddad AF, Lau D, et al. Artificial Intelligence for Adult Spinal Deformity. Neurospine 2019;16(4):686–94.
5. Joshi RS, Lau D, Ames CP. Artificial Intelligence and the Future of Spine Surgery. Neurospine 2019;16(4):637–9.
6. Joshi RS, Lau D, Scheer JK, et al. State-of-the-art reviews predictive modeling in adult spinal deformity: applications of advanced analytics. Spine Deform 2021;9(5):1223–39.
7. Miller EK, Neuman BJ, Jain A, et al. An assessment of frailty as a tool for risk stratification in adult spinal deformity surgery. Neurosurg Focus 2017;43(6):E3.
8. Sciubba DM, Yurter A, Smith JS, et al. A Comprehensive Review of Complication Rates After Surgery for Adult Deformity: A Reference for Informed Consent. Spine Deform 2015;3(6):575–94.
9. Scheer JK, Oh T, Smith JS, et al. Development of a validated computer-based preoperative predictive model for pseudarthrosis with 91% accuracy in 336 adult spinal deformity patients. Neurosurg Focus 2018;45(5):E11.
10. Scheer JK, Osorio JA, Smith JS, et al. Development of a Preoperative Predictive Model for Reaching the Oswestry Disability Index Minimal Clinically Important Difference for Adult Spinal Deformity Patients. Spine Deform 2018;6(5):593–9.
11. Scheer JK, Osorio JA, Smith JS, et al. Development of Validated Computer-based Preoperative Predictive Model for Proximal Junction Failure (PJF) or Clinically Significant PJK With 86% Accuracy Based on 510 ASD Patients With 2-year Follow-up. Spine 2016;41(22):E1328–35.
12. Scheer JK, Smith JS, Schwab F, et al. Development of a preoperative predictive model for major complications following adult spinal deformity surgery. J Neurosurg Spine 2017;26(6):736–43.
13. Durand WM, DePasse JM, Daniels AH. Predictive Modeling for Blood Transfusion After Adult Spinal Deformity Surgery: A Tree-Based Machine Learning Approach. Spine 2018;43(15):1058–66.
14. Safaee MM, Scheer JK, Ailon T, et al. Predictive Modeling of Length of Hospital Stay Following Adult Spinal Deformity Correction: Analysis of 653 Patients with an Accuracy of 75% within 2 Days. World Neurosurg 2018;115:e422–7.
15. Oh T, Scheer JK, Smith JS, et al. Potential of predictive computer models for preoperative patient selection to enhance overall quality-adjusted life years gained at 2-year follow-up: a simulation in 234 patients with adult spinal deformity. Neurosurg Focus 2017;43(6):E2.
16. Ames CP, Smith JS, Pellise F, et al. Development of Deployable Predictive Models for Minimal Clinically

Important Difference Achievement Across the Commonly Used Health-related Quality of Life Instruments in Adult Spinal Deformity Surgery. Spine 2019;44(16):1144–53.

17. Ames CP, Smith JS, Pellise F, et al. Development of predictive models for all individual questions of SRS-22R after adult spinal deformity surgery: a step toward individualized medicine. Eur Spine J 2019;28(9):1998–2011.

18. Pellise F, Serra-Burriel M, Smith JS, et al. Development and validation of risk stratification models for adult spinal deformity surgery. J Neurosurg Spine 2019;1–13.

19. Schwab F, Ungar B, Blondel B, et al. Scoliosis Research Society-Schwab adult spinal deformity classification: a validation study. Spine 2012; 37(12):1077–82.

20. Smith JS, Klineberg E, Schwab F, et al. Change in classification grade by the SRS-Schwab Adult Spinal Deformity Classification predicts impact on health-related quality of life measures: prospective analysis of operative and nonoperative treatment. Spine 2013;38(19):1663–71.

21. Ames CP, Smith JS, Pellise F, et al. Artificial Intelligence Based Hierarchical Clustering of Patient Types and Intervention Categories in Adult Spinal Deformity Surgery: Towards a New Classification Scheme that Predicts Quality and Value. Spine 2019;44(13):915–26.

22. Ames CP, Smith JS, Gum JL, et al. Utilization of Predictive Modeling to Determine Episode of Care Costs and to Accurately Identify Catastrophic Cost Nonwarranty Outlier Patients in Adult Spinal Deformity Surgery: A Step Toward Bundled Payments and Risk Sharing. Spine 2020;45(5):E252–65.

23. Haddad S, Pizones J, Raganato R, et al. Future Data Points to Implement in Adult Spinal Deformity Assessment for Artificial Intelligence Modeling Prediction: The Importance of the Biological Dimension. Internet J Spine Surg 2023;17(S1):S34–44.

24. Safaee M, Lin J, Ames CP. Genetic Age Determined by Telomere Length is Significantly Associated with Risk of Complications in Adult Deformity Surgery despite No Significant Difference in Chronological Age: Pilot Study of 43 Patients. St. Louis, Missouri, USA: presented at: 56th Annual Meeting of the Scoliosis Rsearch Society; 2021.

25. Kaspy MS, Semnani-Azad Z, Malik VS, et al. Metabolomic profile of combined healthy lifestyle behaviours in humans: A systematic review. Proteomics 2022; e2100388. https://doi.org/10.1002/pmic.202100388.

26. Nascentes Melo LM, Lesner NP, Sabatier M, et al. Emerging metabolomic tools to study cancer metastasis. Trends Cancer 2022. https://doi.org/10.1016/j.trecan.2022.07.003.

27. Wu F, Liang P. Application of Metabolomics in Various Types of Diabetes. Diabetes Metab Syndr Obes 2022;15:2051–9.

28. Wishart DS, Feunang YD, Marcu A, et al. HMDB 4.0: the human metabolome database for 2018. Nucleic Acids Res 2018;46(D1):D608–17.

Advancements in Robotic-Assisted Spine Surgery

A. Daniel Davidar, MBBS[a], Kelly Jiang, MS[a], Carly Weber-Levine, MS[a],
Meghana Bhimreddy, BA[a], Nicholas Theodore, MS, MD[a,b,*]

KEYWORDS

• Robotics • Technology

KEY POINTS

• Robotics provides increased accuracy in navigation and screw placement in spinal surgery
• These systems have utility in instrumentation, kyphoplasty, and tumor resection surgical cases, as well as others
• Pitfalls of robotics systems include longer duration of surgical procedures, the need for preoperative planning, and the risk of intraoperative malpositioning

INTRODUCTION

In 1985, Victor Scheinman developed the Programmable Universal Machine for Assembly 200, the first robot used in human surgery, to biopsy brain lesions.[1] In 2004, Mazor Robotics Ltd (Cesarea, Israel) designed the SpineAssist, which was the first robot developed for use in spine surgery.[2] The use of robotics in spine surgery is evolving rapidly, due in part to a favorable learning curve and decreased operative time as surgeons gain experience with robotics platforms.[3,4,5]

The basic intraoperative workflow has remained consistent among most commercially available robots used in spine surgery. In brief, preoperative computed tomography (CT) with 1 mm slice thickness is loaded onto the robot software, allowing the surgeon to plan the screw trajectory preoperatively.[6] The original iteration of the SpineAssist was fixed onto the patient's spinous process or percutaneous frame via Kirschner-wires (K-wires), but newer generations of spinal robots can be affixed to the posterior superior iliac spine or spinous process without a K-wire. Intraoperative fluoroscopic images are merged onto preoperative CT images on the robot, with the assistance of image registration fiducial markers. The robot or robotic arm aligns in position according to the pre-planned trajectory. The initial workflow with the SpineAssist consisted of using the K-wire to confirm trajectory, followed by drilling, introducing a cannulated dilator, and finally threading a guidewire to facilitate screw placement. Current robots have an end effector attached to the robotic arm through which the power drill is introduced, and the screw placement is performed. Newer robots can also utilize intraoperative cone beam CT or even plain radiographs in place of preoperative CT for screw planning.

The areas in which spinal robotics can be applied have steadily expanded, beginning with the lumbosacral region and progressing to the cervicothoracic region and even the brain. In this review, we will discuss advances in spinal robotics, providing an overview of their existing capabilities, advantages, and challenges, as well as considering the possible future directions of robotic spine surgery (**Table 1**).

ROBOT-ASSISTED CERVICAL PROCEDURES

Initial robot-assisted screw placement commonly included thoracic, lumbar, and sacral screws. Cervical screw placement was uncommon, due to concerns regarding the complexity of cervical anatomy and the risk of neurologic injury and

[a] Department of Neurosurgery, Johns Hopkins University School of Medicine, Baltimore, MD, USA;
[b] Orthopaedic Surgery & Biomedical Engineering, Department of Neurosurgery, Johns Hopkins University School of Medicine, Baltimore, MD, USA
* Corresponding author. 600 North Wolfe Street Meyer 7-113, Baltimore, MD 21287.
E-mail address: theodore@jhmi.edu
Twitter: @DrNTheodore (N.T.)

Neurosurg Clin N Am 35 (2024) 263–272
https://doi.org/10.1016/j.nec.2023.11.005
1042-3680/24/© 2023 Elsevier Inc. All rights reserved.

Table 1
Overview of FDA-approved robots for spine surgery

Robot Name, Manufacturer	FDA Approval Year; Indication for Use	FDA-Approved Accuracy (mm)
SpineAssist,[81] Mazor Robotics Ltd	2004; Positioning of surgical instruments during spinal stabilization surgery. Enables preoperative planning and spatial positioning of the surgical tool during procedures.	N/A
Renaissance,[82] Mazor Robotics Ltd	2011; Positioning of surgical instruments or implants during general spinal surgery. Can be used in either open or percutaneous procedures.	N/A
ROSA ONE Spine,[83] Zimmer Biomet	2016; Spatial positioning and orientation of instrument holders or tool guides for standard neurosurgical instruments during spine surgery. Guidance is based on intraoperative plan developed with 3D imaging software. Indicated for posterior lumbar pedicle screw placement.	Robot absolute accuracy: <0.75 Robot repeatability: <0.10 Guidance application accuracy: <2 Navigation accuracy: < 1.5
ExcelsiusGPS,[84] Globus Medical	2017; Intended for locating anatomic structures and spatial positioning of an instrument holder or guide tube for navigating and/or guiding compatible surgical instruments in open or percutaneous procedures. Indicated for placement of spinal and orthopedic bone screws.	N/A
Mazor X Stealth,[85] Mazor Robotics Ltd	2018; Positioning of surgical instruments or spinal implants during general spinal and brain surgery. Can be used in open, minimally invasive, or percutaneous procedures. Mazor X 3D imaging capabilities provide a processing and conversion of 2D fluoroscopic projections from standard C Arms into volumetric 3D image. Mazor X navigation tracks the position of Instruments and Identifies that position on diagnostic or intraoperative images.	≤1.5

(continued on next page)

Table 1
(continued)

Robot Name, Manufacturer	FDA Approval Year; Indication for Use	FDA-Approved Accuracy (mm)
ROSA ONE,[86] Zimmer Biomet	2019; Spatial positioning and orientation of instrument holders or tool guides for standard surgical instruments during spine surgery. Guidance is based on an intraoperative plan developed with 3D imaging software. Intended for thoracolumbar pedicle screw placement.	Robot arm positioning: <0.75 Device applicative accuracy: <2
Cirq Robotic Alignment Module,[87] Brainlab	2020; An accessory to the compatible Brainlab IGS Spinal software for intraoperative image-guided localization to achieve pre-planned trajectories with surgical instruments. Indicated for spinal screw placement.	Positional accuracy: ≤ 2 Trajectory angle: $\leq 2°$

Abbreviations: FDA, food and drug administration; IGS, image-guided surgery; N/A, not available.

vertebral artery compromise.[7] Additional concerns included screw malpositioning, incomplete fusion, pseudoarthrosis, or haloing of screws.[8–10] However, more recently, posterior cervical screws have been placed using robot assistance.[11–14]

Initial studies indicated generally accurate placement of cervical screws with favorable perioperative and postoperative outcomes. A systematic review by Ryan and colleagues analyzed 482 cervical screws placed with robot assistance, among which 379 (78.6%) were pedicle screws.[15] A mean screw deviation of 0.95 mm was reported among 275 screws, and 97.7% of screws were clinically acceptable Grade A or B on the Gertzbein-Robbins scale.[16] In that review, only a single complication of postoperative wound infection was reported. A randomized controlled trial conducted by Fan and colleagues found that although all screws placed were clinically acceptable based on the Gertzbein-Robbins scale, the distribution of Grade A was significantly higher in the group that utilized robot-assisted screw placement compared with the group that used fluoroscopy-guided screw placement.[17] The robot-assisted group also demonstrated decreased mean (interquartile range) screw deviation compared with the fluoroscopy-guided screw placement group (0.83 mm [0.44, 1.29] vs 1.79 mm [1.41, 2.50]; $P < .001$).

Although the placement of C3-7 lateral mass screws is a common procedure, reports of robot-assisted screw placement in the high cervical region are limited. Robot-assisted placements of C1-2 transarticular screws and C2 pars interarticularis screw fixation have been recently described in the literature.[11,14,18,19] In those reports, the intraoperative workflow included the placement of the spinous process registration clamp at C2 for transarticular screws, and at C5 for C2 pars screws. Alternatively, there is a registration array available that can attach directly onto the Mayfield clamp.[19] Robot-assisted surgery can provide increased accuracy during cervical screw placement while avoiding critical neurovascular structures and improving postoperative outcomes.

ROBOTICS IN SPINE TUMOR MANAGEMENT

Spinal tumors are often challenging to treat, as they are difficult to access and often lie in close proximity to critical anatomic structures. Current treatment options for spinal tumors include surgical resection, radiation therapy, or embolization. Robotic approaches have been performed for all 3 of these treatment modalities.

Robot-guided resection for spine tumors is uncommon but has been reported in several case studies. Bederman and colleagues reported using the Renaissance robot system (Mazor Robotics Ltd) for *en bloc* resection of a sacral osteosarcoma.[20] In addition to traditional spine robots, the da Vinci surgical system (Intuitive) has also been used. The da Vinci system consists of 3 or 4 interactive arms attached to a console that provides the surgeon with 3-dimensional, high-resolution cameras, which allow the precise manipulation of the end effectors (eg, scissors, coagulating devices, scalpels) within a closed space, such as the abdominal cavity or the chest. Oh and colleagues reported using the da Vinci system for the resection of presacral tumors in 5 patients.[21] In those patients, the authors found reduced operative time, less blood loss, and shorter length of hospital stay compared with patients who had undergone an open transperitoneal approach. Pacchiarotti and colleagues and Yang and colleagues also reported the use of the da Vinci system in resecting paraspinal schwannomas without significant complications.[22,23] Although the da Vinci robot has been explored in several spinal surgery cases, it can only be used for soft-tissue tasks, is associated with a steep learning curve, and usually requires collaboration with thoracic or general surgeons for efficient use.[24]

Surgical management of spinal tumors often requires vertebrectomy, which is associated with significant morbidity and complex reconstruction.[25] Radiation is an option for many patients, depending on the tumor type and in patients who are not at risk of neurologic compromise. It has become the standard of care for treating skeletal metastases. Radiation can be delivered through external beam radiation therapy or stereotactic radiosurgery (SRS). SRS is delivered via CyberKnife (Accuray Incorporated), a linear accelerator radiosurgery robot with millimeter-level accuracy.[26] This approach is best suited for patients with well-circumscribed tumors, who are not at risk for progressive neurologic decline, and no longer benefit from surgery or traditional radiation.[27] Sahgal and colleagues found that SRS was associated with reduced pain at 3 and 6 months after radiation compared with conventional radiation in a trial of 229 patients.[28] Ryu and colleagues similarly reported complete pain relief after 12 months in 61.3% of patients, with no adverse events after 2 years.[29] In a meta-analysis of retrospective cohorts, Singh and colleagues found that SRS was associated with improved 1-year local control compared with conventional radiation.[30] Although these results are promising, few randomized controlled studies exist, and future studies exploring the optimal radiation dose and fractionation of SRS are needed.

Recent approaches have also focused on less invasive techniques like embolization with Onyx or radiofrequency ablation. Transarterial embolization is the most common approach and is associated with reduced blood loss, but it can be technically challenging due to small vessel size and the risk of spinal cord ischemia.[31] Carefully planned procedures and accurate techniques are therefore critical to reducing complications. The transpedicular approach has been demonstrated in several case studies and may represent a new minimally invasive technique that can leverage the advantages of robotic platforms in the treatment of certain tumors, especially those with increased vascularity.

The ExcelsiusGPS robot (Globus Medical, Inc) has recently been used for the transpedicular embolization of a vertebral hemangioma.[32] This technique allows for simultaneous embolization and pedicle screw placement for fixation. Similarly, the ROSA ONE Spine robot (Zimmer Biomet) has been successfully used for radiofrequency ablation of sacral hemangiomas.[33] Though robot-assisted tumor ablation has only been demonstrated in a handful of illustrative cases, robotic pedicle screw placement has been extensively studied and is associated with increased accuracy and reduced complications. These benefits will likely extend to transpedicular vertebral tumor ablation as it becomes more common.[34]

ROBOT-ASSISTED VERTEBROPLASTY

Vertebral compression fractures are commonly due to osteoporosis and can lead to significant disability and chronic pain.[35] When non-surgical treatments such as medical therapy and braces fail, percutaneous vertebroplasty can be offered. This procedure is generally well tolerated as it is minimally invasive and can provide rapid pain relief, but it requires significant radiation exposure and complications can occur due to low injection accuracy and poor distribution of bone cement.[36] The addition of robotic guidance can assist with preoperative planning. Robotics use is associated with improved outcomes for patients undergoing vertebroplasty, including less bone cement leakage and shorter length of hospital stay compared with fluoroscopy-guided procedures.[37,38] Robotics use may also improve pain management outcomes, though conflicting data have been reported. Jin and colleagues and Shi and colleagues reported Oswestry Disability Index scores favoring fluoroscopy at short-term follow-up, but favoring robot assistance at long-term follow-up.[36,39] Two meta-analyses evaluating pain outcomes after kyphoplasty both reported no significant difference in Oswestry Disability Index or Visual Analog Scale measures of pain between robot-assisted and fluoroscopic approaches.[37,38] Nonetheless, robotics use in kyphoplasty appears to have definitive benefits in reducing cement leakage and hospitalization.

Surgeons also benefit from the integration of robotic systems into kyphoplasty procedures. Robotics use reduces radiation exposure for surgeons by 74% compared with fluoroscopy.[40] And although switching to robot-assisted procedures can require an upfront investment in learning the technique, that learning curve is relatively quick for kyphoplasty procedures, with only 33 cases required to reach 100% accuracy in pedicle cannulation with no significant increase in operative times.[38,41] Currently, nearly all robot-assisted kyphoplasty procedures have utilized the TiRobot or Tianji Robot systems(TINAVI Medical Technologies Co, Ltd), which are only approved for use in China.[37] Adaptation of this procedure to robots approved in the United States may also improve kyphoplasty outcomes for patients and providers alike.

ADVANTAGES OF ROBOT-ASSISTED SURGERY

One of the major goals of robotic surgical systems—especially in the setting of pedicle screw placement—is improved accuracy.[42] Inaccurate screw placement can lead to a variety of consequences, including vascular and neurologic injury that require subsequent revisions. Studies of the SpineAssist showed accurate screw placement as high as 98% in 840 cases.[43,44] Later studies comparing robotic screw placement with a freehand technique, including 2020 and 2023 meta-analyses that looked at 9 and 12 randomized controlled trials, respectively, found improved accuracy with robotic assistance, albeit with some variability between different robotic systems.[45–55] Interestingly, some studies, such as a 2018 meta-analysis of 9 studies, report no difference in accuracy between robotic and fluoroscopy-guided cases.[56,57] Although there are some inconsistencies, increased familiarity with and continued development of robotic systems will further contribute to improved accuracy.

A benefit of robotics systems to both the patient and the surgical team is the significant reduction in radiation exposure in robotic cases compared with conventional fluoroscopic guidance.[44,50–52,54,55,58] For example, Kantelhardt and colleagues found a decrease in x-ray exposure per screw from 77 μSv in conventional cases to 34 μSv in robotic cases.[45] Hyun and colleagues similarly found a 62.5% reduction in radiation when using robotics compared with fluoroscopic guidance.[59] Some earlier studies suggested no change in radiation exposure, but this may have been due to the surgeon's lack of confidence in the accuracy of the robot and request for additional verification imaging.[57,60] Other studies suggest that it is only the surgeon and staff who experience a reduction in radiation exposure, as they can leave the room during the acquisition of intraoperative cone-beam computed tomography.[47] Some studies have shown variations in radiation exposure between different robots. For instance, in a 2020 meta-analysis, Li and colleagues found that surgical procedures conducted with the Mazor robot had reduced fluoroscopy time, whereas those conducted with Tianji and ROSA ONE robots had increased fluoroscopy time when compared with freehand techniques.[60] This finding may be explained by the Mazor robot being the earliest-introduced robot and surgeons having more trust in the system, or it may be due to Mazor utilizing preoperative scans for screw planning rather than intraoperative scans like those used in the other systems.[60] Ultimately, lowering radiation exposure is a priority for both the surgical team and the patient, and is a key consideration in developing surgical approaches. Further studies will need to be done to better define this potential advantage of robotic technology.

Other advantages to robotic surgery include reduced length of hospitalization, as well as decreased adverse events, blood loss, and revision rates.[2,45,55,58,59] In the same 2020 meta-analysis, Li and colleagues found a significant decrease in length of hospital stay in patients undergoing robotic surgeries, especially for degenerative diseases.[60] Other studies evaluating screw placement for thoracolumbar fractures showed no change in the length of hospital stay.[49] In regard to adverse events, robotic cases can have reduced rates of dural tears, cerebrospinal fluid fistulas, and postoperative infections.[45,55,58,61] Studies have also shown a reduction in blood loss in robotic cases,[56,61] which is well explained by the minimally invasive robotic approach, though other studies report no difference in blood loss.[48,49] Finally, in the 2020 Li and colleagues meta-analysis, revision rates were shown to be significantly lower in robotic-assisted surgeries compared with the freehand technique, likely attributable to the improved accuracy of screw placement with the robotic approach.[60] Several other studies similarly found reduced revision rates in robotic-assisted cases.[55] A study considering many of these factors in the cost-effectiveness of introducing robotic surgery into a neurosurgical practice estimated cost savings of over \$600,000 in 1 year of 557 thoracolumbar instrumentation cases.[62]

DISADVANTAGES AND COMPLICATIONS TO ROBOTIC SURGERY

Several important challenges and disadvantages to robotic surgery should be considered. First, the accuracy of the robot relies on the match between the preoperative images and the patient's true anatomy. This match can be affected by several factors, such as the quality of the preoperative image and inaccuracies in registration.[63] A working knowledge of the principles of image-guided surgery is necessary for the adoption of robotic technology into a surgeon's armamentarium.

Another potential factor causing inaccuracy in robotic cases is the attachment point for the robot. The robot can be attached at several points, including the surgical table, the spinous process, and the posterior superior iliac spine.[2,64] Many surgeons prefer the spinous process or iliac spine fixation points, as these allow the robot to follow the movement of the patient.[56] Studies in which the robot is attached to the surgical table—referred to as a *bed mount* system—have shown reduced accuracy in screw placement during robotic cases compared with fluoroscopic guidance cases.[65] The spinous process or iliac spine may indeed be the preferred attachment point, but misalignment can occur if the clamp to the spinous process becomes loose at any point. Some systems use a "surveillance marker," which allows for immediate notification of a loss of accuracy if the reference array has moved.

Misalignment can also occur due to deflection of the drill or tool tip. This can happen when the facet joint has a steep slope on its lateral aspect, as is especially common in degenerative facet joint hypertrophy, causing the tool tip to become deflected or to "skive" off trajectory.[65] The tool's path can also deviate during blunt perforation of overlying muscle and fascia.[65] This potential for tool misalignment must be should be considered by the surgeon when using robotic guidance. Some systems offer immediate feedback regarding tool tip deflection measuring excessive force on the end effector.

Setting up the robot and all of its corresponding equipment may unfortunately increase the overall length of time for the surgery, with multiple studies showing longer surgical durations.[47,48,50–54,57,60] For instance, Kantelhardt and colleagues found an increase in the average time per screw from 52.9 min in conventional cases to 59.1 min in robotic cases, though the difference was not statistically significant.[45] Ringel and colleagues similarly found that the average time for instrumentation was 95 minutes in robotic cases, compared with 84 minutes in fluoroscopic cases.[65] However, some studies showed no significant difference in operative time between robotic and fluoroscopic cases.[58–61] A 2023 meta-analysis showed a reduction in mean screw insertion time with the robotic approach.[61] As surgeons, residents, and operating room teams become familiar with robotic systems, the time required for using robotic systems will continue to decrease.[66] Studies of learning curves have found that 20 to 30 cases are needed for a surgeon to become proficient with using the robotic system, with 1 study demonstrating a decrease in operative time of 4.6 minutes with each successive case.[4] Another systematic review analyzed linear regression results of several studies and found an improvement of 0.10 minutes per screw for each additional screw placed, while operative time improved by 0.24 to 4.6 minutes with each surgery performed.[4,67] Therefore, after the learning curve levels off, surgeons may benefit from a reduction in operating time.

FUTURE DIRECTIONS

Although robotics in spine surgery is currently most commonly used for pedicle screw placement, its applications will continue to expand to other types of spine surgery. One example is in stem cell therapy for degenerative disk disease, where robotics has the potential to aid in the expeditious and accurate placement of cells within the nucleus pulposus.[68] Another example is lumbar spinal injections, which are a common treatment option for people with chronic low back pain. The application of robotics to injections may not only improve accuracy but could also reduce procedure time and minimize the number of insertion attempts. Several different prototypes have been developed using piezoelectric motors under magnetic resonance imaging or fluoroscopic guidance.[69–72] These models have shown improved accuracy over freehand injections in cadaveric and phantom studies, and it is anticipated that future studies in humans will come soon.

Other uses of robotics will be seen in the placement of instrumentation in complex pelvic trauma.[73,74] The ability to fixate these difficult fractures has implications for spinal surgeons, especially in the realm of lumbosacral-pelvic fixation where reconstruction of the spine after tumor resection can be difficult. Utilizing real-time image guidance can significantly improve navigation within these tight corridors and offer spinal surgeons novel fixation techniques for complicated reconstructions.[75]

In addition to the task of placing instrumentation, it is only a matter of time before robotic platforms aid in the bone removal and decompression aspect of spinal surgery. This feature has been part of hip and knee robotic platforms for several years.[76,77] These orthopedic systems allow the surgeon to remove bone using a drill the surgeon controls but that is programmed to stay within a pre-planned volume. This precision allows for the removal of bone and highly accurate placement of prostheses, all while leading to improved outcomes over conventional freehand bone removal.[78] In spine surgery, the bone anatomy is more complicated than in the hips and knees, and the adjacent structures—including the spinal nerves and spinal cord—are far less tolerant to inaccuracy. Nonetheless, robot-assisted bone removal and decompression are being done in the laboratory and will surely be brought into the operating room soon.[78]

Furthermore, the combination of enabling technologies holds great promise. While there has recently been a heightened interest in endoscopic spinal surgery, the learning curve for this technology has been steep. The combination of robotics and endoscopy might aid in the adoption of this technology.[79]

It is evident that there is great potential for robotics in spine surgery in the years to come, with future directions including automation, incorporation of augmented reality, and the possibility for remote spine surgery. With machine learning and artificial intelligence, automation will allow robotic devices to help with surgical planning and learn the surgeon's movements over time to eventually predict and perform the surgical movement while the surgeon oversees the robot.[6] Remote surgery has also been explored, with Tian and colleagues publishing a study on telerobotic spinal surgery successfully placing pedicle screws in 12 patients with the TiRobot system.[80] Although there are obvious risks to telerobotic surgery, it may be especially useful in remote areas with reduced access to experienced spinal surgeons.[59,80]

CLINICS CARE POINTS

- Improved accuracy for screw placement.
- Reduction in radiation exposure.
- Can aid in tumor management.
- Attachment and set-up intraoperatively must not be altered during the course of the procedure.

DISCLOSURES

Nicholas Theodore receives royalties from and owns stock in Globus Medical. He is a consultant for Globus Medical and has served on the scientific advisory board/other office for Globus Medical. The remaining authors have no conflicts of interest to disclose.

REFERENCES

1. Kwoh YS, Hou J, Jonckheere EA, et al. A Robot with Improved Absolute Positioning Accuracy for CT Guided Stereotactic Brain Surgery. IEEE Trans Biomed Eng 1988;35(2):153–60.
2. Lieberman IH, Togawa D, Kayanja MM, et al. Bone-mounted miniature robotic guidance for pedicle screw and translaminar facet screw placement: Part I - Technical development and a test case result. Neurosurgery 2006;59(3):641–50.
3. McKenzie DM, Westrup AM, O'Neal CM, et al. Robotics in spine surgery: A systematic review. J Clin Neurosci 2021;89:1–7.
4. Pennington Z, Judy BF, Zakaria HM, et al. Learning curves in robot-assisted spine surgery: a systematic review and proposal of application to residency curricula. Neurosurg Focus 2022;52(1):E3.
5. Jiang K, Hersh AM, Bhimreddy M, et al. Learning Curves for Robot-Assisted Pedicle Screw Placement: Analysis of Operative Time for 234 Cases. Oper Neurosurg (Hagerstown) 2023;25(6):482–8.
6. D'Souza M, Gendreau J, Feng A, et al. Robotic-Assisted Spine Surgery: History, Efficacy, Cost, And Future Trends. Rob Surg Res Rev 2019;6:9.
7. Klepinowski T, Żyłka N, Pala B, et al. Prevalence of high-riding vertebral arteries and narrow C2 pedicles among Central-European population: a computed tomography-based study. Neurosurg Rev 2021;44(6):3277.
8. Cheung JPY, Luk KDK. Complications of Anterior and Posterior Cervical Spine Surgery. Asian Spine J 2016;10(2):385.
9. Leven D, Cho SK. Pseudarthrosis of the Cervical Spine: Risk Factors, Diagnosis and Management. Asian Spine J 2016;10(4):776.
10. Yoshihara H, Passias PG, Errico TJ. Screw-related complications in the subaxial cervical spine with the use of lateral mass versus cervical pedicle screws: A systematic review. J Neurosurg Spine 2013;19(5):614–23.
11. Kisinde S, Hu X, Hesselbacher S, et al. Robotic-guided placement of cervical pedicle screws: feasibility and accuracy. Eur Spine J 2022;31(3):693–701.
12. Farah K, Meyer M, Prost S, et al. Robotic Assistance for Minimally Invasive Cervical Pedicle Instrumentation: Report on Feasibility and Safety. World Neurosurg 2021;150:e777–82.

13. Su XJ, Lv ZD, Chen Z, et al. Comparison of Accuracy and Clinical Outcomes of Robot-Assisted Versus Fluoroscopy-Guided Pedicle Screw Placement in Posterior Cervical Surgery. Global Spine J 2022;12(4):620.

14. Tian W. Robot-assisted posterior C1-2 transarticular screw fixation for atlantoaxial instability a case report. Spine (Phila Pa 1976) 2018;41:B2–5.

15. Beyer RS, Nguyen A, Brown NJ, et al. Spinal robotics in cervical spine surgery: a systematic review with key concepts and technical considerations. J Neurosurg Spine 2022;38(1):66–74.

16. Gertzbein S, Robbins S. Accuracy of pedicular screw placement in vivo. Spine (Phila Pa 1976) 1990;15(1):11–4.

17. Fan M, Liu Y, He D, et al. Improved Accuracy of Cervical Spinal Surgery with Robot-Assisted Screw Insertion: A Prospective, Randomized, Controlled Study. Spine (Phila Pa 1976) 2020;45(5):285–91.

18. Wang Y, Zeng C, Tian W. Magerl Method of C1-C2 Transarticular Screw Fixation. Navigation Assisted Robotics in Spine and Trauma Surgery 2020;23–30.

19. Sacino AN, Materi J, Davidar AD, et al. Robot-assisted atlantoaxial fixation: illustrative cases. J Neurosurg: Case Lessons 2022;3(25). https://doi.org/10.3171/CASE22114.

20. Bederman SS, Lopez G, Ji T, et al. Robotic guidance for en bloc sacrectomy: A case report. Spine 2014;39(23):E1398–401.

21. Oh JK, Yang MS, Yoon DH, et al. Robotic resection of huge presacral tumors: Case series and comparison with an open resection. J Spinal Disord Tech 2014;27(4).

22. Pacchiarotti G, Wang MY, Kolcun JPG, et al. Robotic paravertebral schwannoma resection at extreme locations of the thoracic cavity. Neurosurg Focus 2017;42(5):E17.

23. Yang MS, Kim KN, Yoon DH, et al. Robot-assisted Resection of Paraspinal Schwannoma. J Kor Med Sci 2010;26(1):150–3.

24. Amin AG, Barzilai O, Bilsky MH. CT-Based Image-Guided Navigation and the DaVinci Robot in Spine Oncology: Changing Surgical Paradigms. HSS J 2021;17(3):294–301.

25. Bandiera S, Boriani S, Donthineni R, et al. Complications of En Bloc Resections in the Spine. Orthop Clin N Am 2009;40(1):125–31.

26. Chang SD, Main W, Martin DP, et al. An analysis of the accuracy of the CyberKnife: a robotic frameless stereotactic radiosurgical system. Neurosurgery 2003;52(1):140–7.

27. Gerszten PC. The Role of Minimally Invasive Techniques in the Management of Spine Tumors: Percutaneous Bone Cement Augmentation, Radiosurgery, and Microendoscopic Approaches. Orthop Clin N Am 2007;38(3):441–50.

28. Sahgal A, Myrehaug SD, Siva S, et al. CCTG SC.24/TROG 17.06: A Randomized Phase II/III Study Comparing 24Gy in 2 Stereotactic Body Radiotherapy (SBRT) Fractions Versus 20Gy in 5 Conventional Palliative Radiotherapy (CRT) Fractions for Patients with Painful Spinal Metastases. Int J Radiat Oncol Biol Phys 2020;108(5):1397–8.

29. Ryu S, Deshmukh S, Timmerman RD, et al. Stereotactic Radiosurgery vs Conventional Radiotherapy for Localized Vertebral Metastases of the Spine: Phase 3 Results of NRG Oncology/RTOG 0631 Randomized Clinical Trial. JAMA Oncol 2023;9(6):800–7.

30. Singh R, Lehrer EJ, Dahshan B, et al. Single fraction radiosurgery, fractionated radiosurgery, and conventional radiotherapy for spinal oligometastasis (SAFFRON): A systematic review and meta-analysis. Radiother Oncol 2020;146:76–89.

31. Ozkan E, Gupta S. Embolization of Spinal Tumors: Vascular Anatomy, Indications, and Technique. Tech Vasc Intervent Radiol 2011;14(3):129–40.

32. Hersh AM, Jin Y, Xu R, et al. Transpedicular Onyx embolization of a thoracic hemangioma with robotic assistance: illustrative case. J Neurosurg: Case Lessons 2023;5(26).

33. Kaoudi A, Capel C, Chenin L, et al. Robot-Assisted Radiofrequency Ablation of a Sacral S1-S2 Aggressive Hemangioma. World Neurosurg 2018;116:226–9.

34. Fatima N, Massaad E, Hadzipasic M, et al. Safety and accuracy of robot-assisted placement of pedicle screws compared to conventional freehand technique: a systematic review and meta-analysis. Spine J 2021;21(2):181–92.

35. Silverman SL. The clinical consequences of vertebral compression fracture. Bone 1992;13(SUPPL. 2):S27–31.

36. Jin M, Ge M, Lei L, et al. Clinical and Radiologic Outcomes of Robot-Assisted Kyphoplasty versus Fluoroscopy-Assisted Kyphoplasty in the Treatment of Osteoporotic Vertebral Compression Fractures: A Retrospective Comparative Study. World Neurosurg 2022;158:e1–9.

37. Zhang Y, Peng Q, Sun C, et al. Robot Versus Fluoroscopy-Assisted Vertebroplasty and Kyphoplasty for Osteoporotic Vertebral Compression Fractures: A Systematic Review and Meta-analysis. World Neurosurg 2022;166:120–9.

38. Chen H, Li J, Wang X, et al. Effects of robot-assisted minimally invasive surgery on osteoporotic vertebral compression fracture: a systematic review, meta-analysis, and meta-regression of retrospective study. Arch Osteoporosis 2023;18(1):1–17.

39. Shi B, Hu L, du H, et al. Robot-assisted percutaneous vertebroplasty under local anaesthesia for osteoporotic vertebral compression fractures: a retrospective, clinical, non-randomized, controlled

study. Int J Med Robot Comput Assist Surg 2021; 17(3):e2216.

40. Barzilay Y, Schroeder JE, Hiller N, et al. Robot-Assisted vertebral body augmentation: A radiation reduction tool. Spine 2014;39(2):153–7.

41. Yuan W, Cao W, Meng X, et al. Learning Curve of Robot-Assisted Percutaneous Kyphoplasty for Osteoporotic Vertebral Compression Fractures. World Neurosurg 2020;138:e323–9.

42. Kia C, Esmende S. Robotic-assisted Spine Surgery: A Review of its Development, Outcomes, and Economics on Practice. Tech Orthop 2021;36(3):272–6.

43. Pechlivanis I, Kiriyanthan G, Engelhardt M, et al. Percutaneous placement of pedicle screws in the lumbar spine using a bone mounted miniature robotic system: First experiences and accuracy of screw placement. Spine (Phila Pa 1976) 2009; 34(4):392–8.

44. Devito DP, Kaplan L, Dietl R, et al. Clinical acceptance and accuracy assessment of spinal implants guided with spineassist surgical robot: Retrospective study. Spine (Phila Pa 1976) 2010;35(24): 2109–15.

45. Kantelhardt SR, Martinez R, Baerwinkel S, et al. Perioperative course and accuracy of screw positioning in conventional, open robotic-guided and percutaneous robotic-guided, pedicle screw placement. Eur Spine J 2011;20(6):860.

46. Yang JS, He B, Tian F, et al. Accuracy of Robot-Assisted Percutaneous Pedicle Screw Placement for Treatment of Lumbar Spondylolisthesis: A Comparative Cohort Study. Med Sci Monit 2019;25:2479.

47. Li C, Wang Z, Li D, et al. Safety and accuracy of cannulated pedicle screw placement in scoliosis surgery: a comparison of robotic-navigation, O-arm-based navigation, and freehand techniques. Eur Spine J 2023;1:1–11.

48. Li C, Li H, Su J, et al. Comparison of the Accuracy of Pedicle Screw Placement Using a Fluoroscopy-Assisted Free-Hand Technique with Robotic-Assisted Navigation Using an O-Arm or 3D C-Arm in Scoliosis Surgery. Global Spine J 2022. https://doi.org/10.1177/21925682221143076/ASSET/IMAGES/LARGE/10.1177_21925682221143076-FIG4.

49. Lin S, Wang F, Hu J, et al. Comparison of the Accuracy and Safety of TiRobot-Assisted and Fluoroscopy-Assisted Percutaneous Pedicle Screw Placement for the Treatment of Thoracolumbar Fractures. Orthop Surg 2022;14(11):2955.

50. Li HM, Zhang RJ, Shen CL. Accuracy of Pedicle Screw Placement and Clinical Outcomes of Robot-assisted Technique Versus Conventional Freehand Technique in Spine Surgery from Nine Randomized Controlled Trials: A Meta-analysis. Spine 2020; 45(2):E111–9.

51. Zhou LP, Zhang RJ, Li HM, et al. Comparison of Cranial Facet Joint Violation Rate and Four Other Clinical Indexes Between Robot-assisted and Free-hand Pedicle Screw Placement in Spine Surgery: A Meta-analysis. Spine (Phila Pa 1976) 2020;45(22): E1532–40.

52. Peng YN, Tsai LC, Hsu HC, et al. Accuracy of robot-assisted versus conventional freehand pedicle screw placement in spine surgery: a systematic review and meta-analysis of randomized controlled trials. Ann Transl Med 2020;8(13):824.

53. Lonjon N, Chan-Seng E, Costalat V, et al. Robot-assisted spine surgery: feasibility study through a prospective case-matched analysis. Eur Spine J 2016; 25(3):947–55.

54. Gao S, Lv Z, Fang H. Robot-assisted and conventional freehand pedicle screw placement: a systematic review and meta-analysis of randomized controlled trials. Eur Spine J 2018;27(4):921–30.

55. Keric N, Eum DJ, Afghanyar F, et al. Evaluation of surgical strategy of conventional vs. percutaneous robot-assisted spinal trans-pedicular instrumentation in spondylodiscitis. J Robot Surg 2017;11(1):17–25.

56. Schatlo B, Molliqaj G, Cuvinciuc V, et al. Safety and accuracy of robot-assisted versus fluoroscopy-guided pedicle screw insertion for degenerative diseases of the lumbar spine: a matched cohort comparison: Clinical article. J Neurosurg Spine 2014; 20(6):636–43.

57. Yu L, Chen X, Margalit A, et al. Robot-assisted vs freehand pedicle screw fixation in spine surgery – a systematic review and a meta-analysis of comparative studies. Int J Med Robot Comput Assist Surg 2018;14(3):e1892.

58. Good CR, Orosz L, Schroerlucke SR, et al. Complications and Revision Rates in Minimally Invasive Robotic-Guided Versus Fluoroscopic-Guided Spinal Fusions: The MIS ReFRESH Prospective Comparative Study. Spine (Phila Pa 1976) 2021;46(23):1661.

59. Hyun SJ, Kim KJ, Jahng TA, et al. Minimally invasive robotic versus open fluoroscopic-guided spinal instrumented fusions. Spine 2017;42(6):353–8.

60. Li J, Fang Y, Jin Z, et al. The impact of robot-assisted spine surgeries on clinical outcomes: A systemic review and meta-analysis. Int J Med Robot Comput Assist Surg 2020;16(6):1–14.

61. Matur AV, Palmisciano P, Duah HO, et al. Robotic and navigated pedicle screws are safer and more accurate than fluoroscopic freehand screws: a systematic review and meta-analysis. Spine J 2023;23(2):197–208.

62. Menger RP, Savardekar AR, Farokhi F, et al. A Cost-Effectiveness Analysis of the Integration of Robotic Spine Technology in Spine Surgery. Neurospine 2018;15(3):216–24.

63. Soriano-Baron HM, Martinez-del-Campo EM, Crawford NP, et al. Robotics in spinal surgery: the future is here. Barrow Quarterly; 2016.

64. Judy BF, Soriano-Baron H, Jin Y, et al. Pearls and pitfalls of posterior superior iliac spine reference frame

placement for spinal navigation: cadaveric series. J Neurosurg: Case Lessons 2022;3(9). https://doi.org/10.3171/CASE21621.

65. Ringel F, Stüer C, Reinke A, et al. Accuracy of robot-assisted placement of lumbar and sacral pedicle screws: A prospective randomized comparison to conventional freehand screw implantation. Spine (Phila Pa 1976) 2012;37(8). https://doi.org/10.1097/BRS.0B013E31824B7767.

66. Judy BF, Pennington Z, Botros D, et al. Spine Image Guidance and Robotics: Exposure, Education, Training, and the Learning Curve. Int J Spine Surg 2021;15(s2):S28–37.

67. Shlobin NA, Huang J, Wu C. Learning curves in robotic neurosurgery: a systematic review. Neurosurg Rev 2022;46(1):14.

68. Silverman LI, Dulatova G, Tandeski T, et al. In vitro and in vivo evaluation of discogenic cells, an investigational cell therapy for disc degeneration. Spine J 2020;20(1):138–49.

69. Li G, Patel NA, Melzer A, et al. MRI-guided lumbar spinal injections with body-mounted robotic system: cadaver studies. Minim Invasive Ther Allied Technol 2022;31(2):297–305.

70. Meinhold W, Martinez DE, Oshinski J, et al. A Direct Drive Parallel Plane Piezoelectric Needle Positioning Robot for MRI Guided Intraspinal Injection. IEEE Trans Biomed Eng 2021;68(3):807–14.

71. Margalit A, Phalen H, Gao C, et al. Autonomous Spinal Robotic System for Transforaminal Lumbar Epidural Injections: A Proof of Concept of Study. Global Spine J 2022. https://doi.org/10.1177/21925682221096625/ASSET/IMAGES/LARGE/10.1177_21925682221096625-FIG6.

72. Gao C, Phalen H, Margalit A, et al. Fluoroscopy-Guided Robotic System for Transforaminal Lumbar Epidural Injections. IEEE Trans Med Robot Bionics 2022;4(4):901–9.

73. Carlson JB, Zou J, Hartley B. Placement of LC-II and trans-sacral screws using a robotic arm in a simulated bone model in the supine position – a feasibility study. J Exp Orthop 2022;9(1):36.

74. Smith AF, Carlson JB. Robotic-assisted percutaneous pelvis fixation: A case report. Clin Case Rep 2023;11(6). https://doi.org/10.1002/ccr3.7527.

75. Liu ZJ, Gu Y, Jia J. Robotic guidance for percutaneous placement of triangular osteosynthesis in vertically unstable sacrum fractures: a single-center retrospective study. J Orthop Surg Res 2023;18(1):8. https://doi.org/10.1186/s13018-022-03489-4.

76. Sugano N. Computer-Assisted Orthopaedic Surgery and Robotic Surgery in Total Hip Arthroplasty. Clin Orthop Surg 2013;5(1):1.

77. Hill D, Williamson T, Lai CY, et al. Robots and Tools for Remodeling Bone. IEEE Rev Biomed Eng 2020; 13:184–98.

78. Liow MHL, Xia Z, Wong MK, et al. Robot-Assisted Total Knee Arthroplasty Accurately Restores the Joint Line and Mechanical Axis. A Prospective Randomised Study. J Arthroplasty 2014;29(12):2373–7.

79. Kolcun JPG, Wang MY. Endoscopic Treatment of Thoracic Discitis with Robotic Access: A Case Report Merging Two Cutting-Edge Technologies. World Neurosurg 2019;126:418–22.

80. Tian W, Fan M, Zeng C, et al. Telerobotic Spinal Surgery Based on 5G Network: The First 12 Cases. Neurospine 2020;17(1):114.

81. U.S. Food & Drug Administration (FDA). Special 510(k) premarket notification. Available at: https://www.accessdata.fda.gov/cdrh_docs/pdf3/K033413.pdf. Accessed July 25,2023.

82. U.S. Food & Drug Administration (FDA). Special 510(k) premarket notification. Available at: https://www.accessdata.fda.gov/cdrh_docs/pdf11/K110911.pdf . Accessed July 25,2023.

83. U.S. Food & Drug Administration (FDA). Special 510(k) premarket notification. Available at: https://www.accessdata.fda.gov/cdrh_docs/pdf15/K151511.pdf . Accessed July 25,2023.

84. U.S. Food & Drug Administration (FDA). Special 510(k) premarket notification. Available at: https://www.accessdata.fda.gov/cdrh_docs/pdf17/K171651.pdf . Accessed July 25,2023.

85. U.S. Food & Drug Administration (FDA). Special 510(k) premarket notification. Available at: https://www.accessdata.fda.gov/cdrh_docs/pdf18/K182077.pdf . Accessed July 25,2023.

86. U.S. Food & Drug Administration (FDA). Special 510(k) premarket notification. Available at: https://www.accessdata.fda.gov/cdrh_docs/pdf18/K182848.pdf . Accessed July 25,2023.

87. U.S. Food & Drug Administration (FDA). Special 510(k) premarket notification. Available at: https://www.accessdata.fda.gov/cdrh_docs/pdf20/K202320.pdf . Accessed July 25,2023.

Moving?

Make sure your subscription moves with you!

To notify us of your new address, find your **Clinics Account Number** (located on your mailing label above your name), and contact customer service at:

Email: journalscustomerservice-usa@elsevier.com

800-654-2452 (subscribers in the U.S. & Canada)
314-447-8871 (subscribers outside of the U.S. & Canada)

Fax number: 314-447-8029

Elsevier Health Sciences Division
Subscription Customer Service
3251 Riverport Lane
Maryland Heights, MO 63043

*To ensure uninterrupted delivery of your subscription, please notify us at least 4 weeks in advance of move.

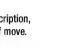

Printed and bound by CPI Group (UK) Ltd, Croydon, CR0 4YY

08/05/2025

01864749-0014